AF706018

Compendium medicine

Pocket
Acute Medicine

Romée Snijders & Veerle Smit
Anique Baten, Demi van Bijlevelt, Carlijn Veldman

Together for Healthcare

Want to know more about Compendium Medicine? Check out our website!

www.compendiummedicine.com

First edition, 2025

© 2023 Compendium Medicine
All rights reserved. Published by Compendium Medicine B.V. under license from Synopsis B.V. as copyright holder. No part of this publication may be reproduced, stored in a computerised database and/or published in any form or in any manner, whether electronic, mechanical, by photocopying, recording or any other means, now known or hereafter invented, without the prior written consent of the publisher.

Neither the publisher nor any authors, contributors, or other representatives of Compendium Medicine assume any liability for any injury and/or damage to persons and property, as a matter of products liability, negligence or otherwise, or from any use or operation of any methods, products, instructions, or ideas in this book. This is a comprehensive limitation of liability that applies to all damages of any kind, including (without limitation) compensatory; direct, indirect, or consequential damages; loss of data, income, or profit; loss of or damage to property and claims of third parties. Links to third-party websites are provided by the publisher in good faith and for information only. The publisher disclaims any responsibility for the materials contained in any third-party website referenced in this work.

This book contains information contained from authentic and highly regarded sources. Every effort has been made to trace copyright holders and obtain their permission for the use of copyright material. Reprinted material is quoted with permission, and sources are indicated. The publisher does not provide medical advice or guidance and this work is merely a reference tool. Healthcare professionals, and not the publisher, are solely responsible for the use of this work including all medical judgments, and for any resulting diagnosis and treatments.

With respect to any pharmaceutical product identified, readers are urged to check the most current information provided on procedures featured by the manufacturer of each product to be administered, to verify the recommended dose or formula, the method, and duration of administration and contraindications. It is the responsibility of practitioners, relying on their own experience and knowledge of their patients, to make diagnoses, determine dosages and the best treatment for each patient, and take all appropriate safety precautions. Compendium Medicine does not accept responsibility or legal liability for any errors in the text, or for the misuse or misapplication of material in this work.

ISBN 978-90-833740-2-4
BISAC MED026000
Thema MKP

MIX
Paper | Supporting responsible forestry
FSC® C118234
www.fsc.org

Preface

Welcome to the *Compendium Community!*

'Together for Healthcare' – these three simple words encapsulate the spirit of our collective mission and underscore the essence of our work. In an era where the complexity of healthcare is becoming increasingly interconnected, collaboration is not merely an option, but an imperative. Our books symbolise the effectiveness of collaboration, knowledge sharing, and a joint commitment to improve and interconnect healthcare.

We proudly present the first edition of our pocket *Acute Medicine* with all the information you want to have at your fingertips. This comprehensive guide is designed to support healthcare professionals embarking on their first hospital out-of-hours shift on the ward, whether they're entering contemplative fields or fast-paced, cutting-edge specialties.

The innovative *Compendium Method*©, designed for medical students and doctors, employs comprehensible illustrations for every medical condition, straightforward tables, icons, and useful mnemonics. It is visually appealing, to the point, and concise. We only focus on the essentials and make sure all the content is comprehensively presented.

Our strength lies in the diverse expertise of our close-knit medical team, consisting of students, doctors, and specialists. This collaborative approach ensures that our content is comprehensive and accurate.

We are committed to inclusivity and aim to make our texts and images a reflection of the diversity of patients our readers provide care to. We aspire for every future doctor and patient to find themselves reflected in our books. Our team works continuously to improve and expand the selection of books. We welcome readers to share their feedback and suggestions, contributing to the continual improvement of our pocket series.

We sincerely wish to express immense gratitude to our team of medical students and healthcare professionals. The outstanding result of their contributions is this extraordinary pocket – a pocket for everybody in healthcare.

Enjoy reading and enjoy working, and we hope to hear from you soon!

Amsterdam, February 2025

Veerle Smit, MD & Romée Snijders, MD
Doctors and founders *Compendium Medicine*

Editorial staff

Want to know more about us?
Scan this QR code.

Editorial board

Romée J.A.L.M. Snijders, MD, PhD & Veerle L. Smit, MD

Chief editor

Gwendolyn Vuurberg, MD, PhD

Pocket editors

Current edition

Demi van Bijlevelt, MD, St Jansdal Hospital, Harderwijk
Carlijn Veldman, MD, Martini Hospital, Groningen

Previous edition

Anique Baten, MD, educational advisor medical training, Radboud University Medical Center, Nijmegen
Carlijn Veldman, MD, Martini Hospital, Groningen

Authors

Current edition

Endry Lim, MD, PhD, MSc, Noordwest Hospital, Alkmaar
Luisa Oliveira e Carmo, MD, OLVG, Amsterdam
Edward Tolpin, BSc, University of Groningen, Groningen

Previous edition

Anique Baten, MD, educational advisor medical training, Radboud University Medical Center, Nijmegen

Acknowledgements

Illustrators

Yente S. Beentjes, MD, University Medical Center Utrecht, Utrecht
Hebe T.A. Boerhout, Utrecht University, Utrecht
Dagmar Bouwer, Leiden University, Leiden
Cas van Cruchten, Maastricht University, Maastricht
Gulizar Durak, Da Vinci College, Dordrecht
Astrid A.H. Feikema, Radboud University, Nijmegen
Dite L.C. de Jong, MD, Elkerliek Hospital, Helmond
Didi D.J. Juin, BSc, University of Applied Sciences, Utrecht
Koen L.C. Ketelaars, MD, GP practice De Brink, Severum
Rosalie C. Krijl, MD, Ask Arbo Artsen, Zeist
Kiki van Langen, University of Amsterdam, Amsterdam
Juliëtte M.E. Linskens, MD, Maastricht University, Maastricht
Kim A.M. van den Nobelen, BSc, Radboud University, Nijmegen
Belle van Rosmalen, University of Amsterdam, Amsterdam
Laura Sanchez, MSc, KU Leuven, Leuven
Carlijn Sturm, BSc, Leiden University, Leiden
Isabel Versmissen, MD, Foundation SBOH, Eindhoven
Linda Xie, MD, Reinier de Graaf Hospital, Delft

Editorial coordinators

Laura M. Barrantes Rodríguez, MD, international relations manager
Pauline Blom, final editor
Vera den Boef, MSc, project manager
Qin-ty Janssen-Bouwmeester, MD, manager diversity and inclusivity
Melanie Goedegebure, project manager
Delano Sanches, MD, BSc, illustration manager

Sounding board

Suzanne Anjie, MD, Noordwest Hospital, Alkmaar
Wytze de Boer, MD, Isala Hospital, Zwolle
Benjamín Fernández Marambio, MD, PhD, Hospital Clínico San Borja-Arriarán, Hospital Clínico Universidad de Chile
Hannah Gillespie, MD, PhD, Newcastle University, Newcastle
Paul Hendriks, MD, PhD, MSc, Erasmus University Medical Center, Rotterdam
Melissa A. van Kuik, MD, OLVG, Amsterdam
Erik Michels, MD, PhD, Amsterdam University Medical Center, Amsterdam
Iris Renken, MD, Radboud University, Nijmegen
Thei Steenvoorden, MD, Amsterdam University Medical Center, Amsterdam
Hitesh Suthar, MD, M. T. Agarwal Hospital, Mumbail
Vicky Tallentire, MD, PhD, University of Edinburgh, Edinburgh

Language support

VVH business translations

Graphic designers

Maria van Doorn, BASc
Ivana Kinkel

Content quality assurance

The editorial board extends its sincere appreciation to the many contributions of doctors, specialists, and professors from around the world who played a pivotal role in crafting this pocket. We wish to express our thanks to the entire international team for their dedicated efforts and invaluable expertise. Special appreciation is also extended to the team of specialists who actively participated in shaping the previous edition.

Current edition

Jelmer Alsma, MD, PhD, Erasmus University Medical Center, Rotterdam
David Baden, MD, PhD, Diakonessenhuis, Utrecht
Jan-Willem H.L., Boldingh, MD, University Medical Center Groningen, Groningen
Prof. Bert-Jan H. van den Born, MD, PhD, Amsterdam University Medical Center, Amsterdam
David Brinkman, MD, PhD, Amsterdam University Medical Center, Amsterdam
Bernard G. Fikkers, MD, PhD, Radboud University Medical Center, Nijmegen
Daisy de Groot, MD, Amsterdam University Medical Center, Amsterdam
Laura van Haaften, MD, Meander Medical Center, Amersfoort
Freek J.H.A. van Hout, MD, Deventer Hospital, Deventer
Prof. Karin Kaasjager, MD, PhD, University Medical Center Utrecht, Utrecht
Geert Kleinnibbelink, MD, PhD, Radboud University Medical Center, Nijmegen
Lisette Langenberg, MD, Erasmus University Medical Center, Rotterdam
Tycho Olgers, MD, University Medical Center Groningen, Groningen
Jose Pedro Cidade, MD, Western Lisbon Medical Center, Lisbon
Suzanne Schol-Gelok, MD, MSc, Albert Schweitzer Hospital, Dordrecht
Robbert W. Schouten, MD, PhD, Amsterdam University Medical Center, Amsterdam
Bas J.J.W. Schouwenberg, MD, Radboud University Medical Center, Nijmegen
Monique Steegers, MD, Amsterdam University Medical Center, Amsterdam
Jan Svihra Jr., MD, PhD, Comenius University, Bratislava
Evelien M. Vermeulen, MD, Amsterdam University Medical Center, Amsterdam
Marieke Visser, MD, PhD, MBA, Amsterdam University Medical Center, Amsterdam
Jeroen Vister, MD, University Medical Center Groningen, Groningen
Prof. André P. Wolff, MD, PhD, University Medical Center Groningen, Groningen
Meta van der Woude, MD, PhD, Amsterdam University Medical Center, Amsterdam
Kadir Yozgatli, MD, Klinikum Links der Weser, Bremen

Previous edition

Jelmer Alsma, MD, PhD, Erasmus University Medical Center, Rotterdam
Ahmad S. Amin, MD, PhD, Amsterdam University Medical Center, Amsterdam
Nettie Arts, Cansius Wilhemina Hospital, Nijmegen
Nilou Ashtiani, MD, co-founder Radiqs and CoMaster
Anouk E.A.T. van Berkel, MD, PhD, Radboud University Medical Center, Nijmegen
Jan-Willem H.L., Boldingh, MD, University Medical Center Groningen, Groningen
Prof. Bert-Jan H. van den Born, MD, PhD, Amsterdam University Medical Center, Amsterdam
Matthias M. Cabri, MD, Amsterdam University Medical Center, Amsterdam
Bernard G. Fikkers, MD, PhD, Radboud University Medical Center, Nijmegen
E.P.L.M. de Gouw, MD, PhD, Radboud University Medical Center, Nijmegen
Laura van Haaften, MD, Meander Medical Center, Amersfoort
Johan van Heel, RN, Radboud University Medical Center, Nijmegen
Nadine Hoonhout, University of Amsterdam, Amsterdam
Freek J.H.A. van Hout, MD, Deventer Hospital, Deventer
Prof. Stephanie C.E. Klein Nagelvoort-Schuit, MD, PhD, Erasmus University Medical Center, Rotterdam
Geert Kleinnibbelink, MD, PhD, Radboud University Medical Center, Nijmegen
Prof. Kees Kramers, MD, PhD, Radboud University Medical Center, Nijmegen
Prof. Mario Maas, MD, PhD, Amsterdam University Medical Center, Amsterdam
Martijn Maas, MD, Dutch Resuscitation Council
Priscilla A. Maria, MD, Founder Inclusive Care
Lars P.W. Mommers, MD, Maastricht University Medical Center, Maastricht/Radboud University Medical Center, Nijmegen
Bregje Neefs, HAN University of Applied Sciences, Arnhem and Nijmegen
Melanie van Pelt-Sprangers, MD, Admiraal de Ruyter Hospital, Goes
Annelies van der Plas, MD, Leiden University Medical Center, Leiden
Cecile J.A. van der Poort, MD, Rijnstate Hospital, Arnhem
Bas J.J.W. Schouwenberg, MD, Radboud University Medical Center, Nijmegen
Charlotte D.C.C. Stolk-van der Heijden, MD, Radboud University Medical Center, Nijmegen
Anouk E. Vermeulen-Putker, MD, Radboud University Medical Center, Nijmegen
Charlotte Vinkenvleugel, MD, manager diversity and inclusivity
Jeroen Vister, MD, University Medical Center Groningen, Groningen
Phillip Voets, MD, PhD, Amphia Hospital, Breda
Thierry X. Wildbergh, MD, Meander Medical Center, Amersfoort
Saskia Willemse, HAN University of Applied Sciences, Arnhem and Nijmegen
Kadir Yozgatli, MD, Klinikum Links der Weser, Bremen

In particular, we thank all medical students, nurses, MD's, PhD's, and medical specialists who participated in the underlying studies.

The Compendium Method©

Manual

In *Compendium Medicine* we use the same concise, visual and schematic description of the various medical specialties. Everything is geared towards overview and structure, facilitating study and practice. We call this the *Compendium Method©*.

Fixed layout

All our medical specialties are presented in the same, recognisable way and each has its own colour and icon. The pockets have a fixed chapter structure. The table of contents of each pocket tells you exactly which topics are covered. The symbols in the corner of the page show what kind of information is being discussed.

- ATLS
- Anatomy
- Physiology
- Patient history
- Physical examination
- Diagnostics
- Treatment
- Differential diagnosis
- Conditions
- Clinical reasoning
- Appendices
- References
- Abbreviations
- Index

Illustrations

The figures provide at-a-glance insight into topics like anatomy or the typical patient. They are also intended for study and practice, such as checking whether you can identify the letters in a picture without looking at the caption.

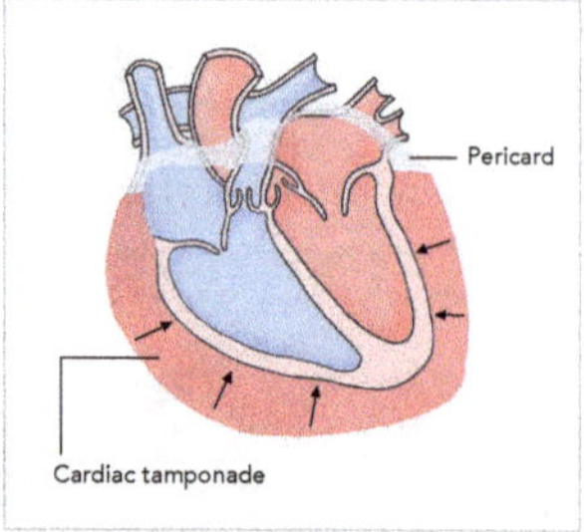

Figure 30 // Cardiac tamponade

Conditions

Each condition in this pocket starts with a full-sentence definition followed by a telegram-style explanation. For each condition, the following icons (as applicable) are discussed. These visual cues that convey specific attributes or features of the condition are also useful when studying. You can cover the text and quiz yourself.

- D Definition
- E Epidemiology
- Ae Aetiology
- R Risk factors
- Hx Patient history
- PE Physical examination
- Dx Diagnostics
- Tx Treatment
  - General
  - Paramedical care
  - Pharmacological treatment
  - Invasive, non-pharmacological treatment
- P Prognosis
- ! Watch out/don´t forget

Tables

We use tables to arrange the information in a clear and structured manner, with columns representing different conditions and rows indicating features or characteristics. Centered formatting for matching features makes it easy to identify similarities and differences.

Diagrams

→ = positive/yes/+ → = negative/no/-

> Diagrams help you reason clinically, starting from a particular symptom, using the green and red arrows as signposts. Always remember that the full differential diagnosis may consist of additional diagnoses.

Fun fact: our founders are Dutch, and in the Netherlands, we refer to a mnemonic as a "donkey bridge". That's why the symbol for mnemonics in our books is a donkey.

Icons & frames

Throughout this pocket you will find highlighted frames.

Tips and tricks	Alarm!	Mnemonic
QR code	Note	Reference to another chapter
Formula	Description of the typical patient	

Punctuation marks

The punctuation in our books also focuses on overview and ensures that the subject matters are covered concisely and effectively.

⊖⊖ Rare	⊕⊕ Most common	↓ Decrease/detoriation
⊖ Uncommon	→ Consequence	♀ Female sex
⊕ Very common	↑ Increase/improvement	♂ Male sex

Abbreviations

We make extensive use of abbreviations, medical terms and symbols for scientific units and quantities. Below are some examples of the abbreviations used in this pocket.

sec	second/seconds	d	day/days	min.	minimum
min	minute/minutes	wk	week/weeks	max.	maximum
h	hour/hours	mo	month/months	e.g.	for example
		y	year/years	L	litre/litres

Index

The pockets include a comprehensive and easy-to-use index. It contains all the topics covered in the books so you can quickly navigate and find the information you are looking for.

Appendices

In the pockets, you will find space for your notes, additional information, reminders, or insights. In addition, handy appendices have been added; these contain specific information that you would like to have at hand and are therefore located at the back of the pockets.

They/theirs

We realise that sex and gender identity are not binary and that there is more variation than just 'woman' or 'man'. For readability's sake (as well as for grammatical reasons) we have therefore chosen to use the pronouns 'they/theirs', regardless of sex or gender identity.

Warning

When studying this pocket, be mindful of the protocols within your own facility and adhere to the established guidelines. It is also essential to understand the circumstances under which you may or may not provide assistance in a given country, as this can potentially have legal consequences.

Want to know more about the Compendium Method©? Scan the QR code.

Table of contents
Acute Medicine

Table of contents
Acute Medicine

Table of contents
Acute Medicine

Care for critically ill patients

In this section, we will provide a general overview of the **primary** and **secondary survey**. The differential diagnosis and treatment of common symptoms is described in more detail in the section *The treatment of a patient with...*

Specific treatment instructions per diagnosis are provided in the section *Conditions*.

Primary survey

General

ABCDE stands for Airway, Breathing, Circulation, Disability and Exposure. Caring for a patient according to the ABCDE system involves the identification and treatment of abnormal vital signs in order of priority. No (prior) diagnosis is required to help the patient! Although the underlying pathology will vary between, for example, the surgical and non-surgical specialisms and each will have a slightly different approach (see Table 1), the essence of the primary survey – acting according to the ABCDE system – is the same.

EMERGENCY SITUATION	METHOD OF CARE
Medical	Systematic approach to medical emergency situations, or care based on the acute internal medicine perspective (MedicALS)
Trauma	Advanced trauma life support (ATLS)
Acute circulatory arrest	Basic life support (BLS) or advanced life support (ALS)
Acute circulatory arrest, paediatrics	Advanced paediatric life support (APLS)
Obstetrics	Managing obstetric emergencies and trauma (MOET)

Table 1 // Various forms of a systematic approach in emergency situations

A reassessment of the ABCDE will be performed to evaluate the effect of any interventions and to provide a systematic record of any changes in the patient's condition. A detailed patient history, including full physical examination and any additional diagnostic tests will only be performed at a later stage, during the secondary survey (see Table 2).

ASSESSMENT	OBJECTIVE
Primary assessment	Stabilisation of the patient achieved through rapid evaluation of vital signs, using the ABCDE approach: treat first what kills first
Reassessment	Repeat assessment to note potential changes and provide a new estimate of the patient's stability
Secondary assessment	Determine the diagnosis by taking an extensive history and performing physical/additional examination, including evaluation of previous procedures

Table 2 // Care for critically ill patient

When a critically ill patient dies, this will always be the result of a failing respiratory or circulatory system, regardless of the underlying condition. The fixed order applied within the ABCDE approach (see Table 3) is based on this fact. In addition to the fact that this system provides support in situations that are generally hectic, it also facilitates the communication within a team and allows for a structured re-assessment of critically ill patients.

Although you may not consider the hospital a high-risk environment, it is still advisable to consider your own safety before assisting a patient. Aspects to consider: needle-stick accidents, risk of contamination, exposure to radiation, etc. In short, handle sharp objects with care, be aware of the potential risk of infection, take hand hygiene measures seriously and err on the side of caution for the use of personal protective equipment (PPE).

<table>
<tr><th colspan="2">ABCDE APPROACH</th></tr>
<tr><td>A</td><td>• Potential cervical spine injury? → immobilise the cervical spine

Look: inspect the mouth and throat → blood/vomit/foreign body/swelling/dentures etc.
Listen: audible respiration/stridor
Feel: if in doubt, feel for air being exhaled

Interventions
• Open the airway by performing head-tilt-chin-lift. N.B.: Jaw-thrust manoeuvre in the case of suspected cervical spine injury!
• Use devices such as oropharyngeal airways (OPA) or nasopharyngeal airways with caution, as the risk of aspiration is high, particularly if the patient is not fully unconscious or when an incorrect size is used. These devices are contraindicated in patients with coagulopathies, suspected basal skull fractures and severe facial injuries. If the patient starts vomiting, quickly turn them on their side.</td></tr>
<tr><td>B</td><td>Look (expose the chest!): external injuries/skin abnormalities/jugular vein distention/central cyanosis/use of accessory breathing muscles/depth and symmetry of thoracic excursions
Listen: hyper-resonant/muffled percussion, breathing sounds, possible adventitious sounds
Feel: position of trachea/subcutaneous emphysema/thoracic instability

Interventions
• Oxygen via non-rebreather mask (NRM), flow rate 12-15L/min, target value saturation 94-98%
• Monitor saturation and respiration frequency
• If necessary, support respiration with non-invasive ventilation (NIV) or ventilation bag
• If the patient shows signs of respiratory insufficiency, consider performing an arterial blood gas (to rule out hypoxaemia, hypercapnia and acute acid-base disorders) and imaging studies (chest X-ray/CT/point of care ultrasonography (POCUS))
• Placement thoracostomy tube by trained specialist</td></tr>
</table>

Table 3A // ABCDE approach

<table>
<tr><th colspan="2">ABCDE APPROACH</th></tr>
<tr><td>C</td><td>Look: internal/external blood loss (chest, abdomen, pelvis, long bones, retroperitoneum), colour/perfusion of the skin
Listen: heart sounds, possible murmurs
Feel: central and peripheral pulsations, assess frequency/regularity/filling. Temperature of extremities.

Interventions:
• Monitor blood pressure (BP), pulse, rhythm, capillary refill time (CRT)
• At least one IV line, preferably two
• Treat shock with fluid resuscitation (500 mL isotonic, warmed crystalloid in 5-10 min) + reassess
• Check for haemorrhage using e-FAST</td></tr>
<tr><td>D</td><td>• Global screening of patient's level of consciousness by means of AVPU and/or Glasgow Coma Scale (GCS). A score of P/U or GCS ≤8 → (potentially) threatened airway.
• Signs of lateralisation
• Pupils: size/shape/symmetry/reaction to light
• Bedside glucose → treat hypoglycaemia: administer 10 g glucose as a slow bolus IV (10 g = 100 mL gluc 10% = 20 mL gluc 50%. Expected increase of 2 mmol/L per 10 g) and check glucose <10 min, repeat if necessary.</td></tr>
<tr><td>E</td><td>• Body temperature
• Complete body inspection (including joints and the patient's backside)
• Cover the patient to prevent hypothermia, unless the patient has severe hyperthermia</td></tr>
</table>

Table 3B // ABCDE approach

In case of catastrophic blood loss:

- 'Treat first what kills first'
- If multiple people present: stop visibly catastrophic heavy bleeding by applying a tourniquet (or plugging wound if possible)
- Be aware of potential bleeding from the chest, abdomen, pelvis and thighs

A Airway

First assess the patient's level of consciousness. A rapid screening using the AVPU score will suffice in this phase of care (see Table 4).

AVPU SCORE	
A	Patient is awake and alert
V	Patient responds only to verbal stimulus
P	Patient responds only to pain stimulus
U	Patient is unresponsive

Table 4 // AVPU score (Alert, Verbal, Pain, Unresponsive)

In patients who only respond to painful stimuli or who are not responsive at all, the level of consciousness is reduced to such an extent that the airway is (potentially) threatened. The airway needs to be cleared and maintained in these patients. If the patient is alert and/or responsive to commands, then one may assume that the patient has a sufficient level of consciousness to maintain their airway without assistance.

> Does the patient have a (potential) injury to the cervical spine? Then measures to immobilise the cervical spine must first be taken. In the event of a (partial) obstruction of the airway, a jaw-thrust manoeuvre (see Figure 1) should be used to open the airway. This will ensure that the cervical spine is manipulated as little as possible.

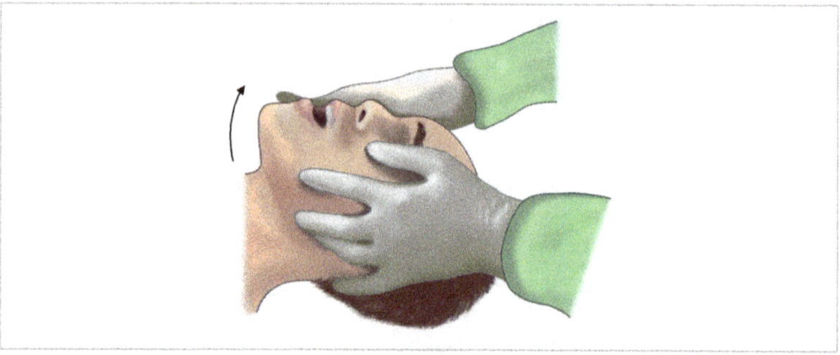

Figure 1 // Jaw thrust

Use a light and a tongue depressor to check the patient's oral cavity for vomit, blood, foreign bodies and swelling of the mucous membranes. Listen for any audible breath sounds (stridor, snoring, expectoration) and/or a hoarse or otherwise abnormal voice. If in doubt, place your wrist/cheek in front of the patient's mouth to feel for a flow of air.

Instead of using a tongue depressor, you can also ask the patient to inhale deeply with an open mouth. This movement raises the pharyngeal arches and flattens the base of the tongue, making a tongue depressor (gag reflex!) unnecessary.

In practice, we distinguish between a partial and a complete airway obstruction. In the case of a partial airway obstruction, the diameter of the airways is restricted, but air can still flow in and out, usually resulting in audible breath sounds (snoring, stridor). Prior to a full respiratory arrest, a complete obstruction of the airways can manifest itself as a paradoxical breathing action; when inhaling, the chest deflates and the abdomen expands and vice versa, in contrast to a normal breathing action in which the chest and the abdomen move in the same direction. Airflow is not observed during paradoxical breathing.

Does the patient have a (partial) airway obstruction? Try to clear the airway by performing a head-tilt/chin-lift manoeuvre (as long as injury to the cervical spine is not suspected) or a jaw-thrust manoeuvre. Additional use of, for example, an OPA/nasopharyngeal airway can be considered, provided you have been trained to use such devices. The risk of aspiration is high, particularly if the patient is not fully unconscious or when an incorrect size is used. However, both these devices are contra-indicated in the event of coagulopathies, suspected basal skull fractures and severe facial injuries.

You should also be aware that neither device results in a secured airway, that these devices will produce varying degrees of effectiveness and that the use of these devices can also result in problems with the airway (e.g. gag reflex → aspiration). In general, you should not attempt a foreign body removal more than once.

An obstructed airway is **always** a medical emergency! Call for help **immediately** in the event of a (suspected) obstructed airway.

See section *The treatment of a patient with an obstructed airway* for practical guidelines.

Clinical deterioration? Always return to A!
Check the effect of your interventions!

B Breathing

Shortness of breath is a very common complaint and is caused by an increased respiratory demand, decreased respiratory capacity or increased subjective demand. Check for external injuries, skin abnormalities, respiration frequency and depth, use of accessory muscles, symmetry of chest excursions, central/peripheral cyanosis and distended jugular veins. Use percussion to examine the chest and check for hyperresonant or muffled percussion. Auscultate the lungs (absent/decreased breathing sounds, wheezing, crepitations, rhonchi). If possible, also listen dorsally, at a later stage if necessary. Consider performing a lung ultrasound. Feel for possible tracheal shift, the presence of subcutaneous emphysema and crepitations/instability upon palpation of the ribs. Also ask the patient if they feel any pain during palpation. Measure the respiration frequency (normally 12-20 breaths per minute) and the oxygen saturation (target value 94-98%). Also evaluate the curve; a low amplitude is indicative of a poor signal and is therefore a less reliable value (e.g. in the case of circulatory shock). Check whether the measured oxygen saturation has been achieved with or without supplemental oxygen. If the patient shows signs of respiratory insufficiency, consider performing an arterial blood gas (to rule out hypoxaemia, hypercapnia and acute acid-base disorders) and imaging studies (chest X-ray/CT/POCUS).

> The pulse oximeter overestimates the oxygen levels in people with darker skin colour.

> If the patient is already receiving supplemental oxygen, do not suspend this when collecting a blood gas sample, but be sure to incorporate this in the interpretation of the results!

Unnecessary use of oxygen at tissue level should be avoided, particularly in the case of reduced supply. Symptoms such as shivering, stress and pain are factors that can result in an undesirable increase in oxygen consumption. Treatment of hypothermia, anxiety and pain can be considered as interventions for the "B" section of the assessment. A simple repositioning of the patient can also produce dramatic results. Oxygenation is reduced in the supine position, particularly in obese patients and patients with pulmonary oedema. Therefore, a seated or semi-upright position is generally preferable for patients experiencing shortness of breath.

Various interventions can be implemented to support the patient's breathing (see Table 5). Start the patient on a NRM at 15 L sooner rather than later and taper this in accordance with the measured saturation values.

Healthcare workers are sometimes incorrectly reticent about administering oxygen to COPD patients, for fear of causing a hypercapnic coma. However, the so-called "hypoxic drive" that forms the basis of a hypercapnic coma occurs in only a small percentage of patients with severe COPD and even these patients have an oxygenation problem that first requires treatment! However, a lower target saturation (88-92%) is applied to these patients after the initial care has been provided, if an initial value is not available.

If a patient has an obvious indication for endotracheal intubation, then this immediately forms a contraindication for use of NIV:

- Circulatory or respiratory arrest
- Non-cooperative/unable to keep airway open or get rid of phlegm
- Severely reduced consciousness
- Acute life-threatening non-respiratory organ failure
- Facial surgery/trauma/deformity
- High risk of aspiration
- Prolonged requirement for ventilation expected
- Recent oesophageal anastomosis

In the event of a reduced respiration frequency (<8/min) and/or insufficient tidal volumes, consider supporting respiration with balloon mask ventilation (Ambu bag). Please note, this is a complex procedure and requires formal training. The two-rescuer technique is often easier to implement by untrained individuals. Call for help, e.g. resuscitation team.

Balloon mask ventilation, two-rescuer technique: doctor places the mask of the balloon mask over the patient's nose and mouth, ensures optimum positioning and opens the airway using the jaw-thrust manoeuvre, whilst instructing the nurse to administer 10-12 breaths per minute. Any dentures that are firmly in position can be left in place, as this facilitates ventilation through an improved seal of the mask on the face.

METHOD OF OXYGENATION AND/OR VENTILATION (least → most invasive)	**MECHANISM**
Nasal cannula	Tube with O_2 supply via two protrusions in the patient's nose
Oxygen mask	Mask with O_2 supply that covers both the nose and mouth
Venturi mask	Mask with O_2 supply that covers both the nose and mouth with the option to adjust the O_2 fraction accurately
Non-rebreather mask (NRM)	Mask with a valve that allows exhaled air to leave the mask, meaning that only the high concentration O_2 from the reservoir is inhaled and to prevent rebreathing of CO_2 (carbon dioxide)
High-flow nasal cannula/optiflow	Tube with two protrusions in the patient's nose, which administer warmed, humidified air with high flow and high FiO_2 whilst generating positive pressure in the airways to keep the airways open
Non-invasive ventilation/ non-invasive positive pressure ventilation (NIV/NIPPV)	Mask that generates positive pressure in the airways to ensure that the airways remain open continuous positive airway pressure (C-PAP)/bilevel positive airway pressure (Bi-PAP)
Larynx mask (invasive)	Supraglottic airway instrument that uses an oropharyngeal cuff to prevent air leakage during positive pressure ventilation. However, the cuff does not provide a complete seal above the vocal cords. Watch out for aspiration.
Intubation (invasive)	The airway is kept open and protected by means of a cuffed tracheal tube in combination with positive pressure ventilation. If intubation fails, the airway must be surgically secured through a tracheotomy.
Extracorporeal membrane oxygenation (ECMO)	ECMO takes over the functioning of the heart and the lungs, with the gas exchange taking place in an artificial lung outside the patient's body

Table 5 // Interventions to support breathing

SpO_2 target value: 94-98% or 88-92% for COPD patients whose initial saturation was not known.

O_2 FRACTION (FiO_2) AND ADMINISTRATION SPEED (APPROX.)	INDICATION
FiO_2 22-45% 0.5-6 L/min	Saturation ↓
FiO_2 50-60% 6-10 L/min (at least 6L/min to prevent rebreathing of CO_2)	Saturation ↓
FiO_2 25-60%, >8 L/min	• COPD flare-up • Other diseases with respiratory insufficiency, for which accurate adjustment of the FiO_2 is important
FiO_2 60-70%, 12-15 L/min	Respiratory insufficiency, first line treatment for conditions with high oxygen requirements (ATLS)
FiO_2 22-100%, 1-60 L/min	• Acute respiratory failure: RR >24/min, paradoxical respiration, use of accessory muscles • Post-extubation stridor • Desire to ventilate without a mask (e.g. in children)
	• Acute respiratory failure: RR >24/min, paradoxical respiration, use of accessory muscles • In COPD patients as alternative for invasive ventilation • Post-extubation with COPD • Cardiac asthma • Immunocompromised patients
FiO_2 21-100%, adjustable	• Brief ventilation in fasting patients • Desire for rapid, invasive ventilation, e.g. during resuscitation • Inability to intubate
	• Insufficient effect of NIV • Acute respiratory failure or exhaustion • GCS <8 (to prevent aspiration) • Upper respiratory tract obstruction
N/A	• Insufficient effect of intubation in prone position • Untreatable air leakage syndromes • Severe untreatable bronchial asthma

See section *The treatment of a patient with dyspnoea* for practical guidelines.

C Circulation

When a patient is said to have a "C problem", this generally refers to shock, an inadequate oxygen supply at the tissue level. The lack of oxygen causes the cells to switch to anaerobic metabolism, which is an ineffective metabolic reaction resulting in increased production of lactic acid as an unwanted by-product.

Closely examine the patient's colour (pale face/feet/hands can indicate hypovolaemia and blood loss, whilst a markedly red face can indicate, for example, vasodilation as a result of underlying sepsis or anaphylaxis). Inspect for external signs of blood loss and check the patency of any drains.

Haemorrhage compartments: blood on the floor, and 4 more
- Chest
- Abdomen/retroperitoneum
- Pelvis
- Thighs/long bone

Evaluate the central venous pressure (CVP) in supine position (distended jugular veins can be a sign of obstructive or cardiogenic shock). Does the patient have a urinary catheter with a urine meter? An output <0.5 mL/kg/h can be an indication of inadequate circulation.

The urine output depends on the patient's weight (mL/kg/h). An average, normal output is 1.5-2 L/d (or 0.5-1.5 mL/kg/h). Oliguria = urine production 100-400 mL/d. Anuria = urine production <100 mL/d. Absolute anuria is suspicious for or due to kidney failure! In that case, check the patency of the catheter tube.

Determine the capillary refill time (CRT). Listen to the heart and assess the rhythm, speed, extra tones and the presence of murmurs. Feel the temperature of the hands and feet (extremities).

The temperature of the extremities is often reduced in the case of hypovolaemic or cardiogenic shock. In the case of distributive shock, the extremities are often warm because of peripheral vasodilation.

Assess the frequency, regularity and strength of (central and peripheral) pulsations. Connect the patient to the monitor and record pulse frequency and cardiac rhythm.

> Rhythm registration does not provide any reliable information about ST-segment deviations. A 12-lead ECG is required for this!

You can set the non-invasive blood pressure measurement (NIBP) to repeat at chosen intervals. This will produce readings for systolic, diastolic and mean arterial pressure (MAP). In practice, blood pressure is generally monitored at intervals of three to five minutes for critically ill patients. Be aware: arrhythmias with a varying follow rate can produce less reliable results due to varying stroke volumes. In such cases, perform manual measurements to rule out any uncertainties.

> Hypotension is a late sign of shock. Young patients are able to compensate for prolonged periods by elevating the heart rate!

Insertion of an IV line is always indicated for critically ill patients, without exception. Choose the largest possible diameter, to allow for volume resuscitation, administration of intravenous (IV) contrast agent and blood collection for labs via the cannula. In practice, two IV lines are often inserted. In addition to allowing for more rapid fluid administration, this also allows simultaneous administration of different medications without concerns about whether or not these products can be administered over the same IV. If insertion in a vein proves unsuccessful, then an intraosseous infusion should be inserted without delay. In that case, contact the emergency response team (ERT) immediately for assistance. Both fluids and medication can be administered via an intraosseous infusion. Blood samples may also be collected, although this should be discussed with the lab beforehand.

The primary objective of performing additional imaging studies (e.g.: chest X-rays, POCUS, echocardiogram, pulmonary CTA) is to determine the underlying cause of the haemodynamic instability. As previously mentioned, the waiting times for these examinations should not result in a delay in performing life-saving procedures. However, during your ABCDE assessment, you can indicate that you are considering a request for additional diagnostic tests as described above, so that the on-call radiologist can be informed about this.

> See the following sections for practical guidelines:
> - The treatment of a patient with chest pain
> - The treatment of a patient with arrhythmia
> - The treatment of a patient exhibiting signs of shock

D Disability

During the assessment of the airway (A), we briefly discussed the AVPU as a fast and reliable method for screening the patient's consciousness. The GCS (see Table 6), also EMV (eye, motor and verbal response) score, is often used for a more detailed assessment. A P/U score on the AVPU corresponds to an EMV score ≤8.

A few rules to ensure correct interpretation of the EMV score:

- Score the best side if signs of lateralisation are observed.
- Always report the specific scores, e.g. E2M2V2 instead of EMV6.
- To classify a motor response as "localisation", the "localising" hand must extend above the clavicle in the case of a painful stimulus to the orbital rim, or the "localising" hand must cross the midline of the body in the case of a painful stimulus to the contralateral hand. If the reaction does move in the direction of the painful stimulus, but does not satisfy these conditions, we refer to this as flexion.
- It is important to distinguish between conscious flexion and pathological flexion (decorticate posturing), which is characterised by flexion of the wrist, abduction of the upper arm and pronation of the forearm.
- In the case of extension (decerebrate posturing), you will observe extreme pronation in addition to extension of the arm.
- We have a tendency to touch the patient when speaking to them. Officially, this is not permitted when assessing a response to a verbal stimulus.

The EMV score was originally introduced and validated for the assessment and follow-up of trauma patients with brain injuries. A correct determination of the EMV score is not that easy, particularly in non-trauma patients. The interpretation of the observations is often open to discussion, which makes a systematic reassessment by subsequent care providers unreliable. It is no coincidence that the AVPU has been included in the (M)EWS instead of the EMV score. Please be aware of this when you use this instrument. Contact the neurologist sooner rather than later if you suspect any underlying neurological pathology.

EYE OPENING	MOTOR RESPONSE	VERBAL RESPONSE
1 No response	**1** No response	**1** No response
2 To pain	**2** Extension response to pain	**2** Sounds
3 To speech	**3** Abnormal flexion response to pain	**3** Words
4 Spontaneously open	**4** Normal flexion response to pain	**4** Confused
	5 Moves to localised pain	**5** Orientated
	6 Obeys commands	

Table 6 // Glasgow Coma Scale

The pupils are checked for (equal) size, shape and response to light. An adequate response is often abbreviated to PEARRL: Pupils Equal and Round, Reactive to Light. An acute severely dilated pupil on one side, in combination with a decreased EMV score, can be attributed to a unilateral space-occupying lesion, such as a haematoma, tumour or abscess. Abnormally constricted pupils on both sides can point to opiate effects or a brain stem infarction. Bilaterally dilated pupils usually occur with sympathetic nervous system stimulation (anxiety, stress, sympathomimetics).

Movements of the extremities (and the face!), as well as the reflexes, are globally assessed for lateralisation. A bedside glucose measurement should be performed immediately for all patients with a reduced level of consciousness or asymmetry in response; hypoglycaemia can mimic numerous neurological presentations.

ABC**DE(FG)**: **D**on't **E**ver **F**orget **G**lucose.

Look specifically for signs of meningeal irritation. If present, this could be indicative of an underlying infection (meningitis) or a subarachnoid haemorrhage (SAH).

The patient must be ABCDE stable before moving on to any procedures, such as a CT of the brain. Therefore, in practice, additional exams such as scans are usually deferred until the secondary survey and the airway is secured (if necessary, by means of intubation) before transporting the patient.

See section *The treatment of a patient with...* for practical guidelines.

E Exposure

The E for Exposure (also called Environment or Examination) can offer clues for an underlying diagnosis, which could help to explain the abnormalities uncovered previously in the ABCD (see Table 1). Inspect the skin closely for abnormalities such as urticaria, erythema, petechiae, blisters, decubitus, etc. It is important that the patient is undressed for this examination and that the back is also inspected.

> If localised skin abnormalities are found, such as with suspected erysipelas, these should be marked at a specific time and reevaluated after a brief period to check for any expansion. To ensure proper hygiene, place a name tag on the pen/marker that was used, and leave this pen with the patient for any further evaluations.

Also closely examine IV insertion sites and any insertion sites of central venous lines and drains. Then take a step back and look at the patient's surroundings. Which IV fluids does the patient have and at which speed is the IV running? Are any medication pumps active, etc.? Feel the temperature/humidity of the skin and look specifically for any abnormal position, swelling or oedema of the extremities. Measure the temperature. A temperature <36°C/96.8°F or >38°C/100.4°F is abnormal and warrants further investigation. Cover the patient again after the examination to prevent cooling.

Secondary survey

The objective of the secondary survey (including medical history, physical examination, additional diagnostic tests) is to identify all signs of illness and injuries of a seriously ill patient. The next step is to create a differential diagnosis, (preliminary) working diagnosis, and corresponding treatment plan.

> If the patient needs to be transported to a different department after receiving initial care, it is important to determine whether additional measures need to be implemented to ensure safe transportation, which materials need to go with the patient and who is most suitable to care for the patient during transportation.

The following pages provide a summary of the medical history and physical examination. See sections on *ECG*, *Radiology* and *Lab values* for more information about additional diagnostic tests.

A few points to consider when assessing an "acute abdomen":

- Be aware that the use of prednisone can mask the clinical signs of an acute abdomen.
- The fact that the diagnostic phase has not been completed yet does not form a contraindication to the administration of analgesia. On the contrary, analgesia will make it easier to perform the physical examination.
- Only a negative D-dimer makes intestinal ischaemia unlikely, a negative lactate does not (an intestine without flow cannot produce lactate).

Handover

Handover between colleagues

Communication tools such as the SBARR/RSVP (see Table 7) are generally used to structure the medical transfer. Use of a standardised transfer method ensures that important information is not forgotten and assists the listener in absorbing the information. It effectively ensures that you speak "the same language".

SBAR	RSVP	EXPLANATION
Situation	**R**eason	• Introduce yourself • Check that you are speaking to the correct person • Identify the patient (who/where) • State the reason for the consultation: what is your query
Background	**S**tory	• Background information regarding the patient • Reason for admission • Relevant past medical history
Assessment	**V**ital signs	• Mention the vital signs systematically (e.g. ABCDE) • Also mention the trends and effects of any interventions
Recommendation	**P**lan	• Mention the conclusion • Formulate your request for assistance explicitly • Verify explicit agreements
Repeat		

Table 7 // SBARR/RSVP

An alternative for SBARR is RSVP:

- **R**eason
- **S**tory
- **V**ital signs
- **P**lan

See Appendix 2 on preparations for handover to the day shift.

Admission

A substantial proportion of the patients who are seen in emergency department (ED) will be admitted to the hospital for treatment/observation. Use the checklist provided below to check all the information thoroughly when preparing such an admission (see Table 8). Then hand over the information in a concise but complete manner to the colleague (nurse/junior (specialist) doctor) who will be taking over the care for the patient.

THEME	SPECIFICATION	EXPLANATION
Nursing orders	Vital signs	• Agree **which** vital signs need to be monitored (Resp, Sat, BP, HR, diuresis, T, MEWS) • Agree **how often** these vital signs need to be checked • Agree which **target values** need to be observed • Agree on the **consequences** that will follow if target values are not achieved
	Lab test	Consider lab tests the following morning and specify which tests need to be performed
	Dietary instructions	NPO/diet (e.g. liquid), etc.
	IV fluids policy	Pump setting/type of IV fluid
	Paramedical professionals	Consider whether support is required from physiotherapy, occupational therapy, dietician, etc. If so, inform the nurse about this, so that these disciplines can be consulted the following day.
	Medication	• State clearly which medication has already been given in ED and at which time • State which medication has been started to treat the working diagnosis • For the patient's home medication, state per product whether this should be continued/suspended temporarily • Consider: antibiotics (prophylaxis), thrombosis prophylaxis, analgesia, PPI, antiemetics, psychopharmaceuticals, sedatives

Table 8A // Admission checklist

THEME	SPECIFICATION	EXPLANATION
Nursing orders	Isolation measures	**Contact isolation (e.g. for diarrhoea)** • Preferably in a single room • Visitors: no specific measures • Healthcare professionals: hand hygiene, disposable apron for potential contact with bodily fluids
		Droplet (contact) isolation (e.g. for vomiting) • Single room • Visitors: FFP1 face mask, hand hygiene after visit • Healthcare professionals: contact isolation + FFP1 face mask
		Strict isolation (e.g. for MRSA) • Special isolation room • Visitors: FFP1/FFP2 face mask (depending on type of micro-organism), PPE (apron, cap, gloves), hand hygiene after removing PPE • Healthcare professionals: hand hygiene, PPE with long sleeves and cap, FFP1/FFP2 face mask (depending on type of micro-organism), hand hygiene after removing PPE
		Airborne isolation (e.g. for (suspected) open tuberculosis) • Special isolation room • Visitors: FFP2 face mask, PPE (apron, cap, gloves), hand hygiene after leaving the room • Healthcare professionals: hand hygiene, PPE with long sleeves and cap, FFP2 face mask, repeat hand hygiene after leaving the room
	Other points of attention	E.g. allergies, required support in home environment (e.g. caring for partner with dementia)
Treatment restrictions	DNR	Do not resuscitate: no resuscitation following circulatory arrest
	No ventilation	No use of ventilator to take over patient's breathing
	No (ICU)	No admission to the Intensive Care Unit (ICU) or the Coronary Care Unit (CCU)
	Other	No surgery, no blood products (e.g. Jehovah's Witness), no dialysis, terminal phase, etc.
Planning discharge	Target date	The time of discharge should be considered from the moment that a patient is admitted. A target date will help the nursing and paramedical staff to make preparations for this discharge.
	Transfer needs	Is the patient expected to return home once discharged? If so, does any (additional) home nursing care need to be organised? Does the patient perhaps need to be transferred to a different care facility?

Table 8B // Admission checklist

Resuscitation

Swift identification of a circulatory arrest, followed by adequate Basic Life Support (BLS) and (in the case of a shockable rhythm) timely defibrillation, are vital to creating the potential for rhythm recovery and associated recovery of the circulation. In this section, we will discuss the principles of basic and specialist resuscitation from the perspective of the novice junior (specialist) doctor.

Many hospitals have their own resuscitation protocol. Although these protocols are based on the current (inter)national guidelines, the details may vary locally. Of course, you should base your actions primarily on the local protocol in your hospital.

BLS covers the basic resuscitation skills. **Immediate Life Support** focuses on the timely detection of a clinical deterioration and starting resuscitation if necessary, then continuing to offer support as a healthcare professional. **Advanced Life Support** covers a set of lifesaving techniques and skills during resuscitation.

This pocket covers the principles of BLS for adults. BLS for paediatric patients differs from that for adults and will not be discussed here.

There is a space at the back of this pocket for you to record the relevant contact details. Write the number of the resuscitation team in your hospital here, so that you will have it with you at all times.

Basic Life Support (BLS)

If a patient is not responding to verbal commands, you should immediately rule out a circulatory arrest. Secure your own safety first (specific measures will depend on the situation) and then approach the patient. Softly shake the patient by the shoulders and ask loudly and clearly: "Are you alright?" (see Figure 2). If the patient does not respond, you must call the emergency number in the prehospital setting. In the hospital setting, a healthcare professional generally checks for the presence/absence of (adequate) breathing, before calling the resuscitation team and (if available) fetching an Automatic External Defibrillator (AED).

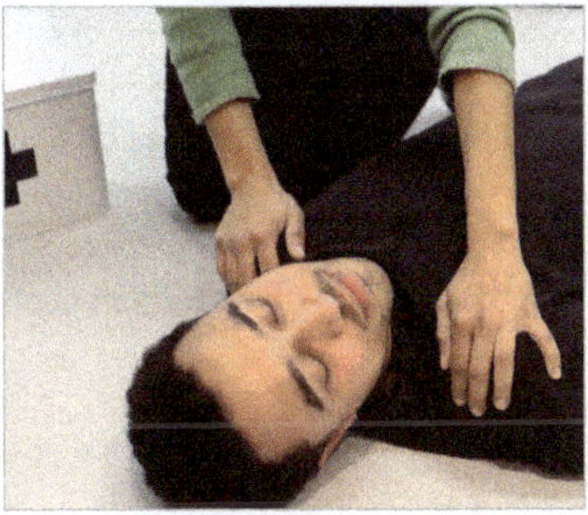

Figure 2 // Initial approach of the patient

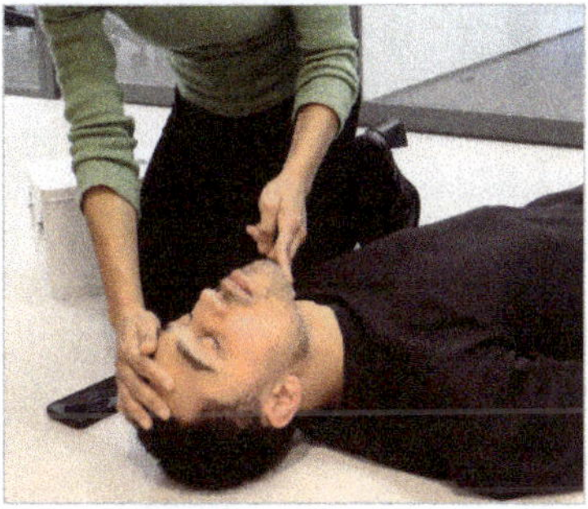

Figure 3 // Opening the airway

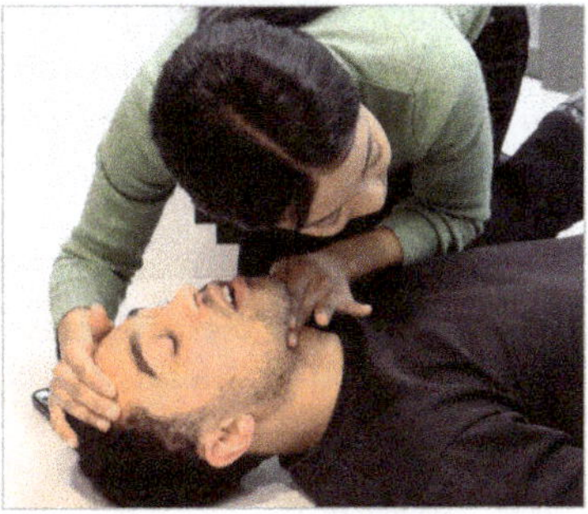

Figure 4 // Observing for signs of life

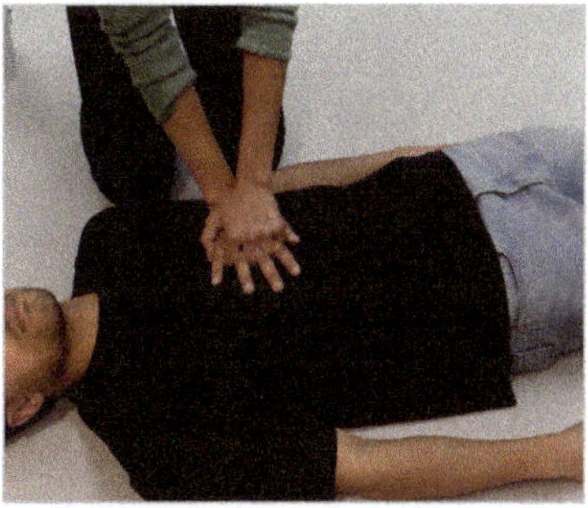

Figure 5A // Chest compressions

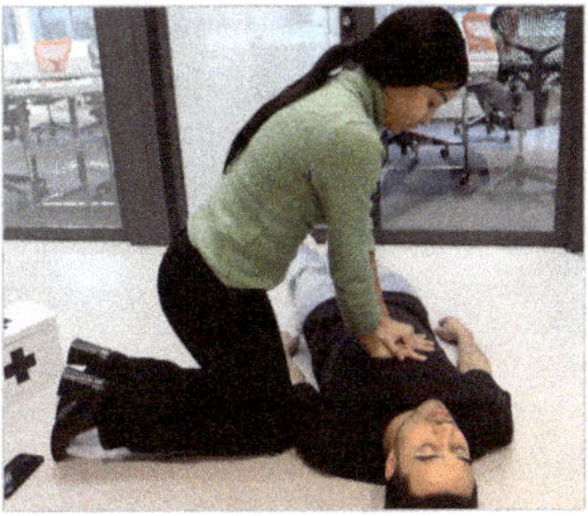

Figure 5B // Chest compressions

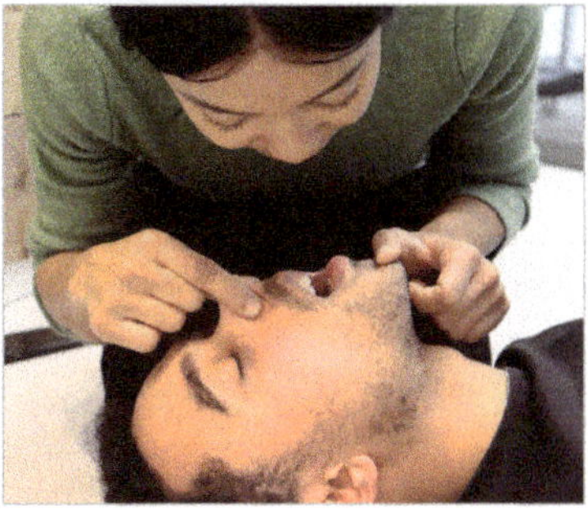

Figure 6 // Ventilation technique during BLS

Many hospitals have AEDs located throughout the hospital. During your introduction period, check whether this is the case in your centre and if so, where the AEDs are located.

Open the airway (see Figure 3). Look for breathing excursions, listen for breathing sounds and feel for exhaled air for a maximum of ten seconds (see Figure 4). If you cannot observe any breathing, or if you are in doubt, start resuscitation. If the patient is lying in a bed, ensure that you create the ideal height for yourself; if you find yourself standing on your toes, lower the bed and/or ask for a stool. Is the patient not in bed, but on the floor? Kneel on the floor next to the patient's chest (see Figure 5).

Place the heel of your one hand in the middle of the sternum and place your other hand on top. Extend your arms, lock your elbows and shift your weight so that your shoulders are in a position that is perpendicular to the patient. Compress the chest. Aim for a depth of 5-6 cm for compressions and a frequency of 100-120/min. Allow the chest to rise fully after each compression. Aim for equal amounts of time for the compression and the relaxation and minimise any interruptions. Chest compressions and rescue breaths should be alternated at a ratio of 30:2.

> A firm surface is essential to ensuring good quality chest compressions. Some hospital beds have a resuscitation setting. A resuscitation board that you can slide under the patient is a good alternative. Both options provide a firm surface that provides sufficient counter-pressure.

Thirty chest compressions are followed by two rescue breaths. Open the airway using the head-tilt/chin-lift, use two fingers of the hand resting on the patient's forehead to seal the nose and calmly blow air in through the mouth (see Figure 6). Aim for an inhalation time of one second and administer just enough volume to allow the chest to rise visibly. Use a pocket mask if available (or, provided you have received formal training, a balloon mask). Some pocket masks have an O_2 port that allows extra oxygen to be administered. When you have a quiet moment, check which materials are available in your centre.

> Bear in mind that proper resuscitation requires a lot of energy. It is therefore preferable to have two healthcare professionals who can swap at least every 2 min, to ensure that the chest compressions remain effective.

See Diagram 1 for a summary of each of the steps in the BLS algorithm. Please note: this describes the prehospital setting. In the hospital setting, as indicated, the healthcare professional at the scene will often first check for breathing, before calling the resuscitation team.

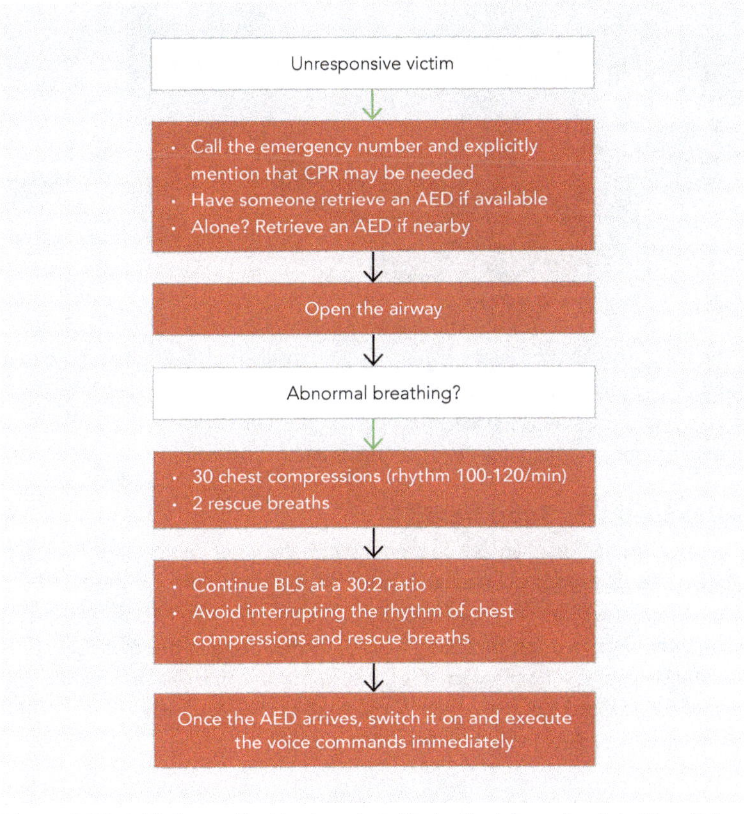

Diagram 1 // Basic Life Support Algorithm. **Important:** this algorithm is for pre-hospital settings. At the hospital, as indicated, the EMT on call will often check the breathing before the CPR team is alerted.

Use the available materials (AED/defibrillator) first at the scene. The self-adhesive defibrillator electrodes can be attached whilst continuing the chest compressions. The electrodes indicate the correct position (see Figure 7).

> If the electrodes won't stick to the chest due to excessive chest hair, remove enough hair to ensure proper adhesion. This is often done in an elective setting, but not typically during acute resuscitation.

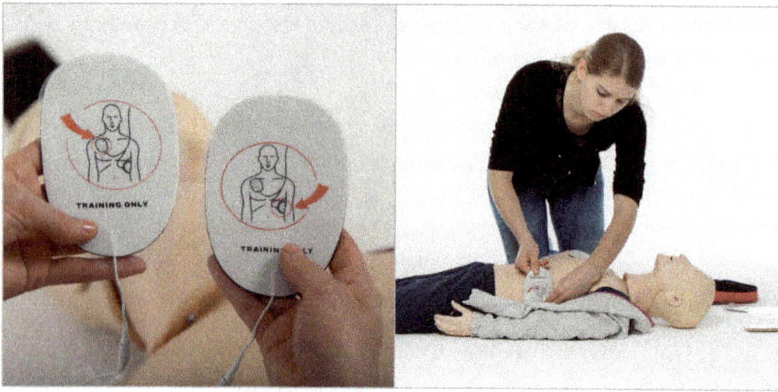

Figure 7 // Positioning of electrodes

When the resuscitation team arrives, continue with your resuscitation attempt until you receive instructions from the team leader. In some cases, AED electrodes that have already been attached can be transferred to the defibrillator, meaning that new electrodes will not be required.

Advanced Life Support (ALS)

The resuscitation team arrives on scene. Whilst the chest compressions are continued, the electrodes will be attached (or if already attached, they will be transferred from the AED to the manual defibrillator after the next AED rhythm check). Check compressions are continued whilst the defibrillator is charging. Only once the defibrillator is fully charged (this takes several seconds) will the team leader give the order to stop chest compressions and to evaluate the cardiac rhythm (see Diagram 2). See Table 9 for the ALS algorithm.

Defibrillation is indicated when a shockable rhythm is detected (ventricular fibrillation (VF) or pulseless ventricular tachycardia (VT)) (see Table 10 // Shockable versus non-shockable rhythms). The circulating team member, who is also responsible for charging the defibrillator, is usually responsible for this important task (and thus the responsibility for ensuring that this is done safely). If a non-shock-able rhythm is detected (pulseless electrical activity (PEA) or asystole), the electrical charge is "dumped". The chest compressions are resumed immediately after defibrillation or dumping of the charge. Ideally, the rhythm check should take no longer than five seconds from start to finish. The effect of the defibrillation and check for a pulse is only evaluated at the next rhythm check, two minutes later.

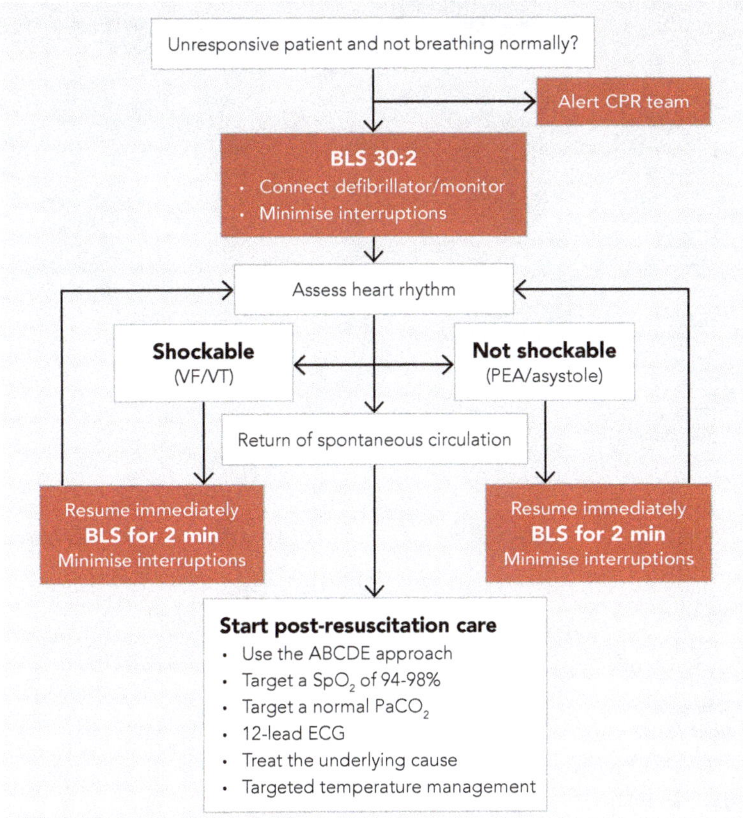

Diagram 2 // Algorithm Advanced Life Support

Force yourself to communicate in a fixed pattern: "Get ready for the next rhythm check. Continue chest compressions. Charge to 200 Joules, remove oxygen." Defibrillator charged: "Stop chest compressions, everybody clear... VF, defibrillating". Or... "Stop chest compressions, everybody clear... this is a rhythm for which I would expect output, dump the charge. Checking for a pulse." Explicitly using words such as "defibrillating" and "dumping" instead of "remove charge" avoids confusion amongst team members and creates a safe working environment. The addition "remove oxygen" applies as long as the patient is not intubated.

DURING CPR	TREAT REVERSIBLE CAUSES (4 H'S AND 4 T'S)
• Give high-quality chest compressions (mechanical chest compressions where possible) • Rotate staff providing compressions to maintain the quality of chest compressions • Administer supplemental oxygen • Use capnography • Start uninterrupted chest compressions after advanced airway interventions • Vascular access (IV/intraosseous) • Give adrenaline every 3-5 min • Give amiodarone after 3rd shock block • Ultrasound: POCUS/transthoracic echocardiogram (TTE) • Consider diagnostics for underlying cause (e.g. coronary angiography (CAG), CT) • Consider extracorporeal membrane oxygenation (ECMO)	Reversible causes of resuscitation setting (4 H's and 4 T's) • Hypoxia • Hypovolaemia • Hypo-/hyperkalaemia/metabolic • Hypothermia/hyperthermia • Thrombosis (coronary or pulmonary) • Tension pneumothorax • Tamponade (cardiac) • Toxins

Table 9 // Algorithm Advanced Life Support

RHYTHM	SAMPLE STRIP	FEATURES	TREATMENT
Ventricular fibrillation	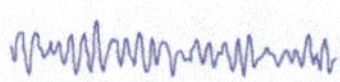	• Irregular wave pattern • QRS complexes cannot be distinguished • Random frequency and amplitude	Shock
Monomorphic ventricular tachycardia	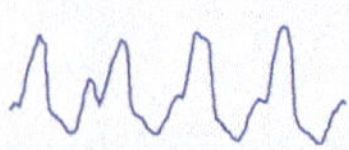	• Wide complexes • Rapid frequency • Constant QRS morphology (monomorphic) versus varying QRS morphology (e.g. Torsades des pointes)	Shock
Polymorphic ventricular tachycardia	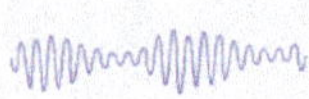		
Pulseless electrical activity	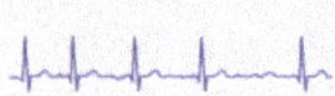	• Clinical manifestation circulatory arrest • Rhythm for which output is expected, but no output is observed	No shock
Asystole	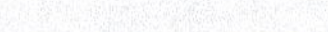	• Absence of ventricular (QRS) activity • Atrial activity (P-peaks) can be present • Rarely a straight line	No shock

Table 10 // Shockable versus non-shockable rhythms

> Sometimes a patient will go into circulatory arrest whilst connected to the monitor ("witnessed arrest"). If a defibrillator is within reach, you can proceed with defibrillation immediately. Once the circulatory arrest has been confirmed, administer a maximum of three shocks in short succession (three-shock strategy). If an organised rhythm is visible on the monitor, check the output. If the patient does not have an organised rhythm, immediately administer the next shock. After the third shock, start BLS if the patient's rhythm has not been restored and evaluate the rhythm again after 2 min. In this case, the three consecutive shocks are viewed as the initial rhythm check and thus as the start of the first block. If defibrillation is taking too long for a "witnessed arrest", start BLS immediately and follow the standard protocols.

The BLS techniques must always be performed properly during the resuscitation. Although the team is jointly responsible, the task of monitoring this is primarily to the team leader. In addition, IV access (intraosseous access, if necessary) must be achieved and the airway should be secured, if possible. Lastly, the end-tidal CO_2 ($etCO_2$) can provide valuable additional information regarding, for example, the quality monitoring of the BLS and the timely detection of the recovery of circulation (see Table 11).

RHYTHM	EXAMPLE
Ventilated patient, intact circulation	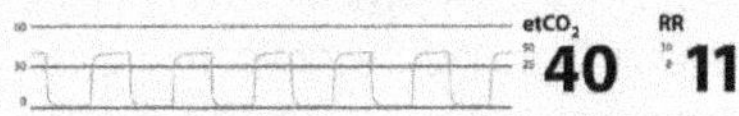
Capnography after intubation. No CO_2 measurable: suspected oesophageal intubation. Remove tube and resume bag valve mask ventilation.	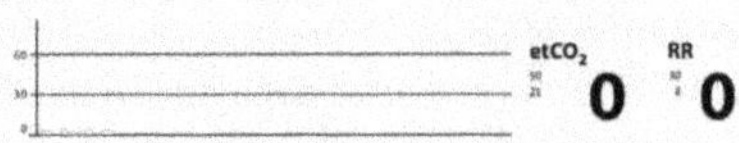
Correctly positioned tube and high-quality chest compressions	
Low $etCO_2$: check BLS quality, watch out for fatigue! Optimal BLS is an indication of poor prognosis.	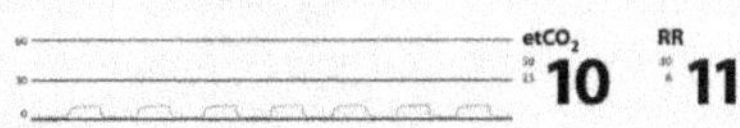
$EtCO_2$ evolution at ROSC	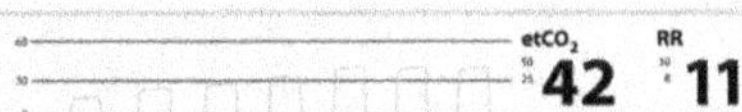
Disconnection	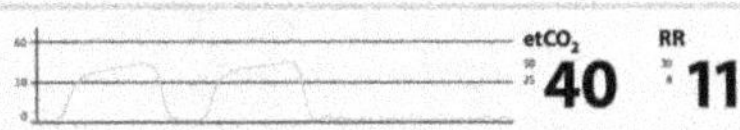

Table 11 // Interpretation $etCO_2$. RR, Respiration rate; ROSC, Return of spontaneous circulation. Please note: $etCO_2$ displayed in mmHg. Use an online calculator to convert the values to kPa if desired.

The $etCO_2$ refers to the CO_2 concentration in the exhaled air, which is measured at the end of the exhalation (normal value 35-45 mmHg or 4.7 to 6.0 kPa).

An electrical shock to restore the cardiac rhythm is not only used as an intervention during resuscitations. The (supra)ventricular arrhythmias can also be treated by administration of a shock, referred to as **cardioversion**. The major difference is that these shocks are administered **synchronously** and usually at a lower energy. In this case, synchronously means that the shock is "synchronised with the R wave". If the shock is administered simultaneously with the T-peak, there is a risk of inducing VF. Most defibrillators are set to asynchronous as the default setting, so that they can be used immediately during a resuscitation. This means that the device must **explicitly** be set to synchronous when treating (supra)ventricular arrhythmias!

Medication ALS algorithm

Adrenaline and amiodarone are administered at set points within the ALS algorithm (see Diagram 3). Adrenaline is a sympathomimetic drug that stimulates the alpha and beta receptors of the sympathetic nervous system. The alpha-adrenergic effect causes vasoconstriction, which improves the perfusion of the myocardium and the brain during chest compressions. Amiodarone is a membrane-stabilising anti-arrhythmic drug, which prolongs the duration of the action potential and the refractory period in the atrial and ventricular myocardium. Flush thoroughly after each administration (fluid bolus of at least 20 cc). This ensures that the medication is actually absorbed in the (limited) central circulation.

In the case of **adrenaline**, following the first administration, the adrenaline needs to be repeated every other block (1 mg adrenaline IV or IO every 4-5 min). The following applies for amiodarone: first administration after the 3rd shock. When administering adrenaline in the context of a three-shock strategy, the initial block consisting of a maximum of three consecutive shocks is considered as one block. This does not apply to **amiodarone**. In the situation where the maximum of three consecutive shocks are administered in the three-shock strategy, amiodarone must be administered immediately after this block.

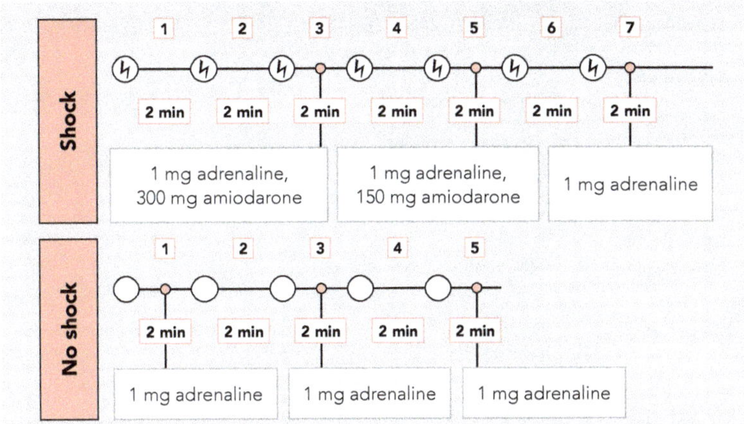

Diagram 3 // Medication ALS algorithm for circulatory arrest, if no interim change in protocol occurs/resuscitation in the form of three-shock strategy has not been started. Adrenaline: administer once → repeat every second block. Amiodarone: first administration after the 3rd shock.

> If return of spontaneous circulation is suspected during one of the resuscitation blocks, the next administration of adrenaline should be postponed until after the rhythm check (due to the risk of inducing arrhythmias). If the next rhythm and pulse check rules out the return of circulation, then the postponed adrenaline should be administered after all.

Reversible causes

The circulatory arrest may be attributed to a reversible cause. These causes are summarised in practice at the four Hs and four Ts. A limited examination, including lab and POCUS, is performed during the resuscitation to check for these underlying causes and treat if necessary (see Table 12).

OBSERVATION	POINTS OF ATTENTION	INTERVENTION
Hypoxia	• Low saturation prior to circulatory arrest • Signs of airway obstruction prior to circulatory arrest	• Ensure that the airway is clear • Administer 100% oxygen
Hypothermia	• Less likely in hospitalised patients • Measure the temperature as centrally as possible	Treat with effective warming techniques (heated infusions, Bair Hugger) and consider warming via ECMO

Table 12A // 4H4T

OBSERVATION	POINTS OF ATTENTION	INTERVENTION
Hypovolemia	• Check the patient's history for signs of blood loss, dehydration, etc. • Signs of blood loss: "blood on the floor and four more" (chest, abdomen, pelvis, legs) • Check any drains that are present	• Treat bleeding • Fluid challenge, if necessary
Hyperkalaemia/ hypokalaemia	• Rapid determination of electrolytes via blood gas • Check most recent lab results	Treat any abnormalities, e.g. administer calcium gluconate and glucose/insulin if patient is found to be hyperkalaemic
Tamponade	• Echocardiogram (during rhythm check) • Keep this in mind particularly after chest trauma or cardiothoracic surgery	Treat by means of pericardio-centhesis and/or thoracotomy
Thrombosis	• Check the patient's history for coronary artery disease/DVT/pulmonary embolism • Swollen calves • Echocardiogram (during rhythm check), look for signs of right ventricular overload	Trombolysis or trombectomy after ROSC if trombolysis un-succesful
Toxins	Check patient's history for suspected/sus-picious exposure	Administer targeted treatment, if possible
Tension pneumothorax	• Symptoms: unilaterally decreased breath-ing sounds, asymmetrical chest move-ments, chest injuries, subcutaneous emphysema, tracheal deviation • Check position of tube, if present	Needle thoracocentesis and/ or thoracostomy, followed by chest drainage

Table 12B // 4H4T

Recently, 5Cs have been added to the list of reversible causes:
- **C**erebral causes (e.g. acute subarachnoid haemorrhage)
- **C**ardiomyopathy (e.g. infectious, dilated, hypertrophic)
- **C**onduction abnormalities
- **C**ongenital abnormalities
- **C**ommotio cordis

Following the administration of IVT, the resuscitation must be continued for 30-90 min before the definitive decision can be made to stop the resuscitation. Consider the use of an automated CPR device.

Post-resuscitation treatment

If any organised electrical activity is observed during the rhythm check, the patient should be monitored closely for signs of ROSC (Return of Spontaneous Circulation), such as palpable pulsations and a significant increase in the $etCO_2$. Once ROSC has been confirmed, you should officially switch to post-resuscitation treatment (see Diagram 4).

Unfortunately, many resuscitation attempts prove unsuccessful. Ideally, the team should make a joint decision to stop resuscitation. Once the resuscitation has been discontinued, the patient should be observed for at least 5 min before confirming death (absence of central pulsations, absence of heart sounds, possibly also asystole on continuous ECG/absence of contractile activity on echocardiogram, absence of pupillary response and corneal reflexes, absence of motor response to painful stimuli). The time at which these criteria are met is recorded as the time of death.

Points of attention for the assessment of the airways and breathing
Return of circulation does not automatically result in return of breathing. Support the patient's breathing as long as necessary. Hypoxaemia and hypercapnia both increase the risk of a new circulatory arrest and secondary brain damage. In the case of a traumatic resuscitation, immobilise the cervical spine until it has been cleared. Insert an NG tube to decompress the stomach. Request a chest X-ray to check the positioning of the endotracheal tube, search for rib fractures, signs of aspiration, etc. The patient should preferably be extubated as soon as possible after they start breathing spontaneously. The stress of coughing caused by the inserted tube can cause further arrhythmias. If the patient is not breathing adequately after ROSC, then the patient should be sedated and intubated.

Points of attention for assessment of the circulation
Ensure continuous monitoring, as the rhythm is not stable so soon after resuscitation. Request a cardiac ultrasound to rule out cardiac tamponade if the patient has elevated CVP/soft heart sounds. Collect blood samples for extensive lab tests; electrolyte imbalances are commonly observed after resuscitation and can result in (potentially avoidable) arrhythmias.

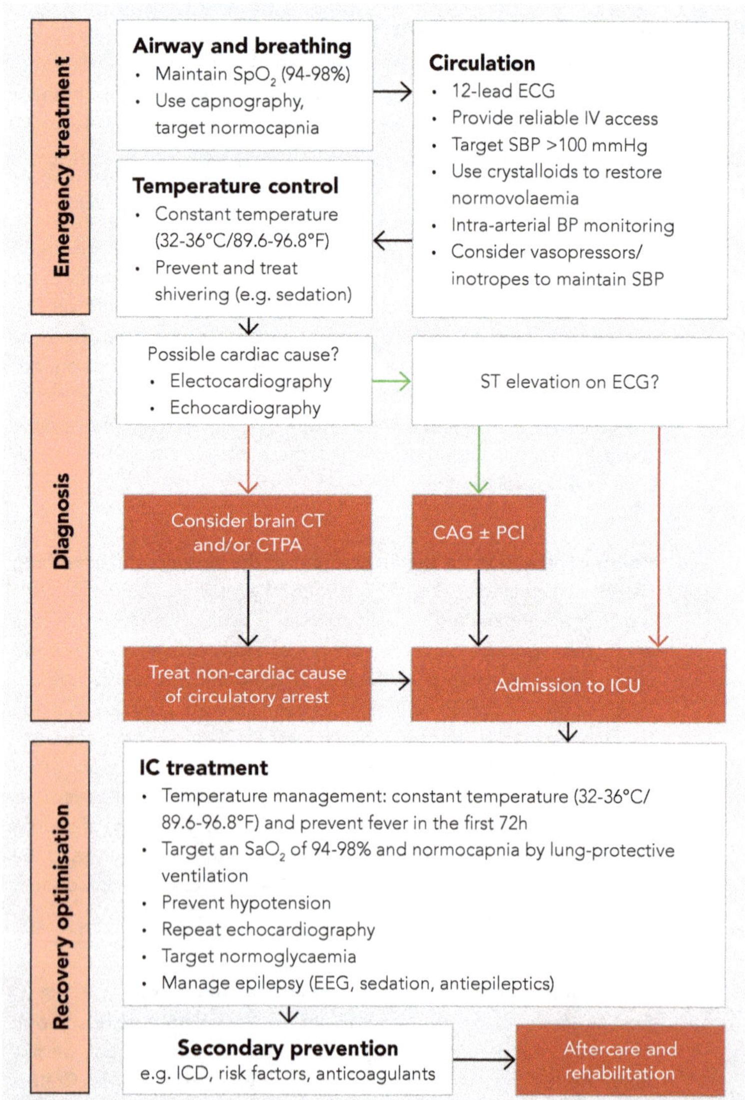

Diagram 4 // Flowchart resuscitation setting
SBP, systolic blood pressure; PCI, Percutaneous coronary intervention; CAG, Coronary angiography; CTPA, Computed tomography pulmonary angiography; IC, intensive care; EEG, electroencephalography; ICD, Implantable cardioverter defibrillator

The post-resuscitation phase is often complicated by the so-called **post-circulatory arrest syndrome**: brain damage, myocardial dysfunction, systemic ischaemia/reperfusion response and the continuation of the underlying pathology. The severity of this syndrome will vary based on the duration and the cause of the circulatory arrest.

Special circumstances

Occasionally you will be involved in resuscitation attempts for which other measures, in addition to the ALS algorithm, need to be implemented to ensure a successful conclusion of the resuscitation. Examples of such situations include resuscitation following drowning, high-energy trauma, electrocution or resuscitation of pregnant women. Very few healthcare professionals will encounter these situations during their career. Do you expect to encounter such special resuscitations regularly in your field? In that case you should complete a certified ALS training course in one of the training centres in preparation for your work.

Resuscitation in the hospital

The boundary between BLS and ALS is less obvious in the hospital than in – for example – the prehospital setting. It is more of a continuum. Sometimes patients will be on a ward with healthcare professionals who are highly trained in recognising and treating a circulatory arrest and there will be no need to call the resuscitation team. However, sometimes a situation may be very similar to the prehospital setting, for example when a visitor (or healthcare professional) collapses in the central hall of the hospital. In that case, bystanders can start the resuscitation and the resuscitation team will take over upon arrival. In order to ease communication, make sure to clear the room of everyone who is not contributing to the resuscitation. Following the initial care, these patients often need to be moved to facilitate an efficient (continuation of the) resuscitation.

Approx. 80% of in-hospital resuscitations are preceded by a deterioration in vital signs. Timely detection of this deterioration, using the MEWS, and subsequent effective intervention can potentially prevent the need for resuscitation.

For more information on responding to emergencies in an out-of-hospital setting, see the pocket *First Aid*.

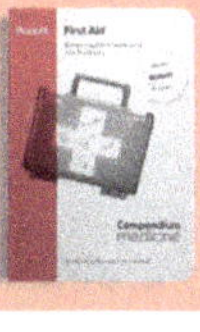

Patient history

Introduction
- Introduce yourself
- Check personal details
- Assess the patient: acute or non-acute, determine reason for consultation and/or chief complaint, nonverbal communication

→

Patient history
- General patient history
- History of presenting complaint/ current illness
- History of relevant system (full review of systems if necessary)

→

Concluding
- Summarise your findings
- Patient's remarks and/or questions
- Explain physical examination and/or indicated diagnostics

Consider psychosocial variables such as language barriers, cultural differences between patients and physicians, financial backgrounds, and addiction, which may impact disease progression.

Diagram 5 // Patient history

An extensive patient history is part of the secondary survey, after the patient has been assessed via the ABCDE approach and has been stabilised.

General patient history

Medical history including past surgeries, medication use (exact dosage, frequency, last dose, administration form), history of substance use (smoking, alcohol, drugs), allergies (latex, plasters, medication, contrast agents), family history, psychosocial history, travel history, social history (home situation, work, study, social support), vaccinations, ill individuals in immediate vicinity.

The mnemonic **AMPLE** can help to remember to ask key questions in acute situations

A: Allergies
M: Medications currently used
P: Past illness/pregnancy
L: Last meal
E: Events/environment related injury

Review of systems

General system

General well-being, itching, fever, chills, night sweats, appetite, weight change (deliberate/unintended), fatigue, exercise tolerance.

> Watch for red flags/B symptoms (e.g. disabling fatigue, weight loss, unexplained fever, night sweats, itching, icterus). These symptoms may be associated with a serious condition, such as malignancy.

Circulatory system

Dizziness/light-headedness (orthostatic), chest pain (on exertion or at rest), palpitations (e.g. fluttering, pounding, racing), dyspnoea (e.g. dyspnoea on exertion or at rest, orthopnoea), nycturia, intermittent claudication, cold extremities, peripheral oedema.

Respiratory system

Dyspnoea (e.g. dyspnoea on exertion or at rest, orthopnoea), acute or chronic onset, coughing (dry, sputum, nocturnal, haemoptysis), audible breathing (e.g. wheezing, rhonchi), chest pain (e.g. worsens when breathing deeply), sputum (e.g. consistency, colour, blood). ENT: sore throat, earache, tinnitus, voice (hoarse), recurrent respiratory infections.

> Dyspnoea caused by a decompensated heart worsens with exertion and when lying down (orthopnoea).

Digestive system

Vomiting (e.g. frequency, blood), nausea, reflux, regurgitations, swallowing problems, abdominal pain, stool pattern (e.g. frequency, consistency, colour, blood or mucus, tenesmus), flatus, icterus, diet, appetite changes.

Urogenital system

Miction (e.g. dysuria, stranguria, haematuria, pollakiuria, polyuria), incontinence, flank pain, changes in bowel habits, sexual history. ♀: vaginal discharge, menstrual cycle, hot flashes. ♂: weak stream, feeling of incomplete emptying, dribbling, discharge, erectile dysfunction, testicular pain or swelling.

Endocrine system

Changes in bowel habits (e.g. diarrhoea/constipation), polydipsia, polyuria, menstrual irregularities, agitation/inertia, cold or heat intolerance, exophthalmos, enlarged thyroid, muscle problems, skin/hair changes, sweating, oedema, weight changes, mood swings, alterations in libido or sexual function.

Locomotor system

Warmth, redness, swelling, cramps, restless legs, joint pain, joint instability, morning stiffness, loss of function, action radius, muscle atrophy.

Haematology system

Bone pain, epistaxis, haematomas, heavy menstrual bleeding, prolonged bleeding, petechiae lymph node swelling, night sweats, fever, fatigue.

Central nervous system

Concentration difficulties, amnesia, dizziness (spinning sensation), loss of consciousness, seizures, headache, impaired senses (e.g. hearing, smell, taste, vision), language, speech, mastication, swallowing, diplopia, abnormal sensation (e.g. numbness, tingling), loss of strength, gait disorders, balance problems, tremors or involuntary movements, psychiatric symptoms.

Skin and mucous membranes system

Skin rash (efflorescence, redness), skin discolouration, nail/finger abnormalities, itching.

Mental health system

Cognitive functioning, sleep problems, anxiety, depression, mood swings, delusions, hallucinations, suicidal thoughts or self-harm.

Acute symptoms

Chest pain

Duration of pain (e.g. long, short, continuous/intermittent), radiation/referred pain (e.g. arm, shoulder, back, epigastric region, and/or jaw), effect of physical exertion (on exertion or at rest), effect of posture, associated symptoms (e.g. dysautonomia, nausea, diaphoresis, palpitations), type of pain (e.g. tearing, oppressive, burning, dull, stabbing), alleviating factors (nitroglycerin spray).

Palpitations

Onset and ending (e.g. sudden/gradual), duration of palpitations (e.g. long, short, continuous/intermittent), regular/irregular, fast/slow, location of palpitations (e.g. throat, chest), medication use, loss/near-loss of consciousness, provoking factors, presence of chest pain, dyspnoea.

Syncope

Onset (e.g. sudden onset, with prodromes), duration of loss of consciousness, recovery (e.g. quick, confusion, slow, recurrence of syncope), triggers (e.g. emotions, coughing, standing up, micturition), associated symptoms (e.g. dysautonomia, palpitations, chest pain, nausea, tremor/shaking limbs, incontinence, lateral tongue bite), skin colour (e.g. red, pale), symptoms afterwards (confusion, neurological deficits, headache), alcohol/drug use, medication use.

Dyspnoea

Duration (acute/subacute/chronic), effect of physical exertion (dyspnoea on exertion or at rest), presence of orthopnoea, relation with inspiration and expiration, fever, recurrent infections, use of antibiotics, associated respiratory symptoms (upper respiratory tract symptoms, cough, sputum, haemoptysis), associated cardiac symptoms (chest pain, palpitations, syncope, diaphoresis), peripheral oedema.

Abdominal pain

Onset (acute/subacute/chronic), localisation of pain, type of pain (e.g. colic, tearing, stabbing), duration (continuous or intermittent), radiation, effect of posture, nausea, vomiting, diaphoresis, stool (consistency, presence of blood or mucus, colour, odour), chest pain.

The essential components of a pain history can be recalled using the mnemonic **SOCRATES**.

Pain (SOCRATES)
Site
Onset (sudden/gradual)
Character (dull, sharp, stinging)
Radiation
Associated symptoms
Time course/duration
Exacerbating, relieving factors (urge to move, pain during transport)
Severity

Physical examination

The next chapter provides a systematic guide to performing a general physical examination. Emphasis is placed on the importance of clear communication and patient comfort throughout the examination. The most important aspects of the general examination are presented.

> This physical examination is part of the secondary survey, after the patient has been assessed via the ABCDE approach and has been stabilised.

Introduction
- Permission (explain examination and consent)
- Wash your hands and use PPE
- Privacy
- Expose target body part

→

Physical examination
- General inspection
- Vital signs (and radial sigs)
- Target physical examination
- Tract-specific examination

→

Concluding
- Thank patient
- Dispose of PPE and wash your hands
- Summarise your findings
- Explain indicated diagnostics and/or next steps

Diagram 6 // Physical examination
PPE, personal protective equipment

General inspection

Gender, age (biological vs. calendar), state of consciousness, mental state, posture, skin colour (e.g. pale, cyanotic, flushing/blushing, icteric), mobility, grooming, nutritional status (e.g. cachexia, BMI), and any medical equipment attached to the patient or in the bedspace.

> Skin colour may give an indication of underlying conditions. For example:
> - Pale → anaemia
> - Cyanosis → hypoxaemia
> - Flushing/blushing → hormonal status, anaphylaxis
> - Icteric → high bilirubin levels

A grey or pale skin colour is often present in patients in shock or who have a syncope, vagal reaction, or acute coronary syndrome.

Anthropometric data

Abdominal circumference, weight, height, BMI.

Vital signs

REFERENCE RANGES					
RR	15-20/min	**Systolic BP**	100-140 mmHg	**T**	36-38°C/ 96.8-100.4°F
SpO_2	>95%	**Diastolic BP**	60-90 mmHg	**CRT**	<2-3 sec
HR/pulse rate	60-100/min	**CVP**	R 4-9 cm H_2O (3-8 mmHg)		

Table 13 // Normal values vital signs (Vx)
BP, blood pressure; CRT, capillary refill time; CVP, central venous pressure; HR, heart rate; RR, respiratory rate; SpO_2, oxygen saturation; T, temperature

A CRT >3 sec suggests poor peripheral perfusion (e.g. hypovolaemia, sepsis, congestive heart failure (HF)).

The first sign of a critically ill patient is increased respiratory rate. Pathophysiology: perfusion ↓ → metabolic acidosis → respiratory compensation (CO_2 ↑ and pH ↓).

Pulse

- Heart rate: 60-100/min
- Heart rhythm: regular or irregular rhythm (e.g. atrial fibrillation, atrioventricular blocks)
- Pulse character/pulse force: full, normal, weak, absent/non-palpable
- In emergency situations or when access to the radial artery is challenging, the carotid pulse can be palpated for assessment

Pulsus paradoxus is a 10 mmHg drop in systolic blood pressure with inspiration and can be palpable at the radial pulse when this difference exceeds 15-20 mmHg. It is suspect for cardiac tamponade, but can also be present in severe pulmonary embolism, severe obstructive lung disease, haemorrhagic shock, or tension pneumothorax.

MEWS

The MEWS (modified early warning score) is an objective parameter for early recognition of patients who are at risk of rapid deterioration (see Table 14). Different hospitals have different trigger scores for notifying physicians: verify that your facility uses the same point assignments listed here.

	+3	+2	+1	0	+1	+2	+3
RR (per min)		<9		9-14	15-20	21-29	≥30
Saturation (%)	<92	92-93	94-95	>95			
Supplemental O_2		Yes		No			
Temperature		<35°C/ <95°F		35.0-38.4°C/ 95-101.1°F		≥38.5°C/ 101.3°F	
Systolic BP (mmHg)	≤70	71-80	81-100	101-199		≥200	
HR (per min)		≤40	41-50	51-100	101-110	111-129	≥130
Consciousness (AVPU score)				Alert	Responds to voice	Responds to pain	Unresponsive

Table 14 // MEWS
AVPU, alert verbal pain unresponsive; BP, blood pressure; HR, heart rate; RR, respiratory rate

> Other variants of the MEWS score may be used at your hospital.

General physical examination

> Make sure you always perform the physical examination in the same order to ensure you do not forget anything. For example you can work from top to toe.

> Always perform the physical examination based on the patient's specific complaints and clinical history. Consider indications or any red flags for additional diagnostics. This chapter provides a focused exploration of the most common general and system-specific aspects of physical examination rather than attempting to cover all aspects comprehensively.

Head and neck

Inspection

Shape/symmetry, carotids, lymph nodes, oral cavity (e.g. corners of mouth (rhagades)), thyroid, trachea.

Auscultation

Carotid bruit (e.g. carotid stenosis).

Palpation

Pulsation carotid artery, lymph nodes, thyroid (e.g. at rest/when swallowing), trachea (i.e. in midline).

Thorax

Lungs

Inspection

Skin abnormalities (e.g. thoracic scars, rash, peripheral and central cyanosis), breathing pattern (e.g. depth, rate, sound, posture, accessory breathing muscles, rhythm, asymmetry in the expiratory and inspiratory phases), chest wall deformities (e.g. asymmetry, pectus carinatum, pectus excavatum, hyperexpansion/barrel chest), extremities (e.g. colour, clubbed fingers, nail clubbing), respiratory effort.

Palpation

Thoracic excursions, epigastric angle, local point tenderness, vocal fremitus, subcutaneous emphysema.

Percussion

Air resonance (normal), dullness (increased tissue density, e.g. pneumonia, pleural effusion), stony dullness (e.g. pleural effusion), hyper-resonance (increased air, e.g. emphysema, pneumothorax), symmetry, lower lung border, shifting lung borders, lung-liver border, diaphragm.

Auscultation

Breathing sounds (vesicular/normal, bronchial/harsh-sounding (e.g. consolidation)), quiet/reduced breath sounds (e.g. silent chest in COPD), symmetry, vocal resonance (volume), inhalation/exhalation ratio, abnormal breath sounds (fine end-inspiratory crackles indicating opening of obstructed central bronchi, coarse crackles indicating opening of distal airways, pleural rub, rhonchi, inspiratory/expiratory stridor, wheezing, muffles or absent breath sounds).

Heart

Inspection

Skin abnormalities (e.g. thoracic scars, rash, petechiae/Osler's node/Janeway lesion/splinter haemorrhages (e.g. endocarditis stigmata)), neck veins (pulsations, CVP ↑), peripheral pitting oedema.

Palpation

Apex beat (heaves/thrills), thrill/vibration.

Percussion

Heart borders (top, left, right).

Auscultation

Heart rate, heart sounds (S1 and S2), S2 splitting, presence of S3 (e.g. in athletes or pathological cause, e.g. post-myocardial infarction, mitral regurgitation, ventricle septum defect, dilated cardiomyopathy) and/or S4 (decreased ventricular compliance, e.g. in hypertrophic cardiomyopathy, aortic stenosis), heart rhythm (regular or irregular, breathing-based or unrelated to breathing), murmurs (timing in systole or diastole, high/low frequency, loudness, radiation over carotid arteries, valve locations, see Figure 8 and Table 15), pericardial friction rub.

> Percussion and palpation play a relatively minor role in respiratory and cardiovascular examination and are not frequently utilised in clinical practice.

VALVE DEFECTS	PHASE OF HEART CYCLE	SHAPE	PMI	ILLUSTRATION
Aortic valve regurgitation	Diastole	Decrescendo	3 ICS left	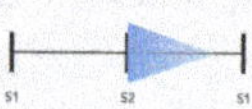
Aortic valve stenosis	Systole	Crescendo-decrescendo	• 2 ICS right • Radiation: carotid artery	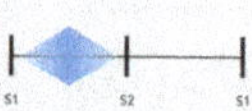
Mitral valve regurgitation	Systole	Holosystolic	• Apex • Radiation: left flank and axilla	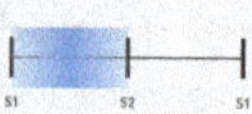

Table 15A // Characteristics of cardiac murmurs caused by valve defects
ICS, intercostal space; PMI, point of maximum intensity

VALVE DEFECTS	PHASE OF HEART CYCLE	SHAPE	PMI	ILLUSTRATION
Mitral valve stenosis	Diastole	Opening snap, presystolic murmur	Apex	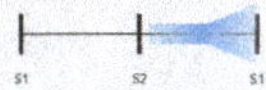
Pulmonary valve regurgitation	Diastole	Decrescendo	2 ICS left	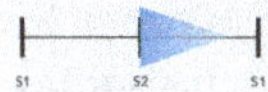
Pulmonary valve stenosis	Systole	Crescendo-decrescendo	2 ICS left	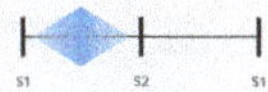
Tricuspid valve regurgitation	Systole	Holosystolic	4 ICS left	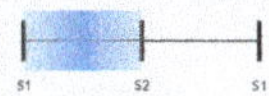

Table 15B // Characteristics of cardiac murmurs caused by valve defects

Abdomen

Inspection

Shape/symmetry (e.g. flanks, swelling, abdominal distension: fat, fluid, flatus, faeces, fetus, fulminant mass), skin abnormalities (e.g. scars, striae, rash, discolouration, caput medusae), abdominal hernias, navel, visible peristalsis.

Auscultation

Bowel sounds (normal, absent, tinkling indicative of mechanical bowel obstruction), bruits (e.g. abdominal aorta aneurysm, renal artery stenosis).

Percussion

Quality (e.g. dull sounds, resonant sounds), organs (e.g. bladder contours, liver contours, spleen contours), pain, shifting dullness (when suspect ascites).

Palpation

Superficial palpation: tenderness, voluntary guarding, involuntary guarding/rigidity (e.g. peritonitis).
Deep palpation: rebound tenderness (e.g. peritoneal irritation), organomegaly (i.e. liver/spleen), masses (e.g. location, size, shape, consistency, mobility), organs (i.e. aorta, bladder, colon, gallbladder, liver, spleen, kidneys).

> Perform a rectal examination e.g. if there is suspicion of gastrointestinal bleeding. Other examinations not discussed in this pocket: external genitalia (e.g. to rule out testicular torsion as a cause of referred abdominal pain or an indirect inguinal hernia).

Extremities

Inspection

Hair growth, skin abnormalities (e.g. scars, rash, bruises), contours of arms and legs (e.g. muscle atrophy), symmetrical spacing between extremities and torso, joints (e.g. redness, position, swelling), oedema, trophic disorders (e.g. shiny skin, lack of hair, brittle nails), varicose veins.

Palpation

Peripheral oedema (e.g. pitting, non-pitting), arterial pulsations (i.e. brachial, radial, femoral, popliteal, posterior tibial, dorsalis pedis arteries, see Figure 9), reflexes (i.e. biceps, brachioradialis, triceps, quadriceps muscles, achilles tendon), sensation, temperature, swelling, joint (e.g. range of motion (ROM), stiffness, stability), muscles (e.g. tonus, tenderness, eccentric and concentric strength).

> Always assess peripheral circulation in the acute or cardiologic patient: capillary refill time (sternum), warm/cold extremities, and strong/weak peripheral pulsations.

Nervous system

Mental status

GCS (see Table 6), cortical functions (attention, orientation, speech, language).

Cranial nerves

Pupils (size, symmetry, pupillary response), eye tracking (diplopia, nystagmus), Donders' test (visual field defects), facial sensory and motor function (hypesthesia, facial nerve palsy), hearing (Rinne, Weber), tongue motor function (deviation), pharyngeal arches, strength tests trapezius and sternocleidomastoid muscles.

Motor exam

Muscle tone, pronator drift, Mingazzini sign, strength tests individual muscles extremities.

Sensory exam

Light touch, sharp/dull discrimination, vibration sense, joint position sense, sense of movement.

Coordination exam

Romberg test, tandem gait test, finger to nose test, finger to finger test, heel to shin test.

Reflexes

Biceps reflex, triceps reflex, knee reflex, Achilles reflex, plantar response, abdominal skin reflex.

Gait exam

Stride width and length, arm movements, tiptoe and heel walking.

Meningeal irritation

Neck stiffness, Kernig's sign, Brudzinski's sign.

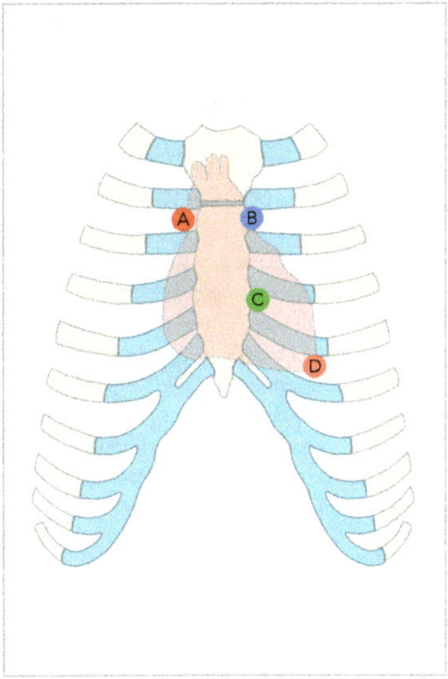

Figure 8 // Location of PMI of valvular murmurs
A: Aortic valve **B:** Pulmonary valve **C:** Tricuspid valve **D:** Mitral valve

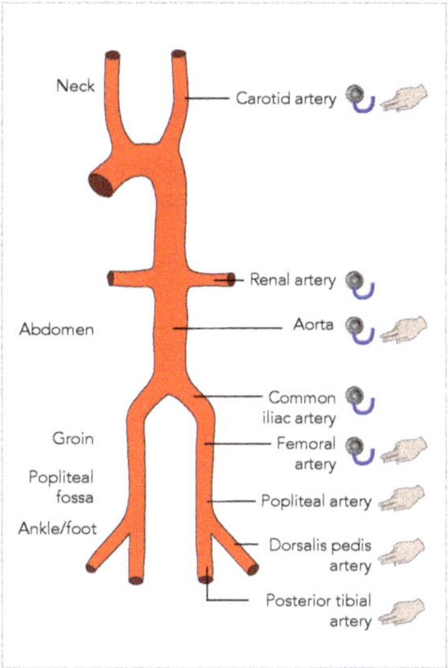

Figure 9 // Palpation arterial pulsations

Diagnostics

Lab values

Reference values may vary between laboratories. Test results should preferably be compared to previous values. Request them from the patient's general practitioner (GP) or another hospital if necessary. While the following section provides examples of conditions associated with altered lab values, it is essential to acknowledge that the scope of medical diagnoses is vast and varied.

When interpreting laboratory results, it is crucial to consider them in the context of all findings. For example, an isolated thrombocytopaenia has a completely different differential diagnosis than thrombocytopaenia with anaemia and leukopaenia (pancytopaenia).

General blood count

LAB VALUE	EXPLANATION	INTERPRETATION
Haemoglobin (Hb)	Protein in erythrocytes that can bind and carry oxygen	↑ Polycythaemia: • Primary polycythaemia: - Congenital - Acquired: malignant bone marrow disease • Secondary polycythaemia: - Secondary to hypoxia: e.g. COPD or smoking, sleep apnoea, high altitudes, right-to-left shunts, congestive HF - Secondary to kidney disease - Secondary to EPO-producing tumour - Secondary to alcohol use disorder ↓ Anaemia, see Table 17
Haematocrit (Ht)	Measure of red blood cell volume in relation to total blood volume	↑ • Dehydration • Primary or secondary polycythaemia ↓ Anaemia

Table 16A // General blood count

CMV, cytomegalovirus; COPD, chronic obstructive pulmonary disease; DIC, disseminated intravascular coagulation; EBV, Epstein-Barr virus; EDTA, Ethylenediaminetetraacetic acid; EPO, erythropoietin; HIV, human immunodeficiency virus; ITP, immune thrombocytopenia; HELLP, haemolysis, elevated liver enzyme levels and low platelet levels

LAB VALUE	EXPLANATION	INTERPRETATION
Mean corpuscular volume (MCV)	Measure of the average volume of erythrocytes, see Table 17	↑ Macrocytic = Normocytic ↓ Microcytic
Platelet (PLT) count	• Platelets/thrombocytes • Are primary haemostasis by aggregation	↑ Thrombocytosis: • During/after infection/inflammation • Splenectomy/hyposplenism • Iron deficiency • Myeloproliferative disease • Paraneoplastic ↓ Thrombocytopenia: • Synthesis ↓: bone marrow insufficiency, e.g. tumour invasion/medication-induced, deficiencies (vitamin B12, folic acid), liver disease (e.g. liver cirrhosis), hyperthyroidism/hypothyroidism • Utilisation/degradation ↑: disseminated intravascular coagulation (DIC), sepsis, immune thrombocytopenia (ITP), medication-induced immune thrombocytopenia, post-transfusion, preeclampsia/HELLP, viral infection (e.g. CMV, EBV, hepatitis B/C, HIV), parasitic infection (malaria), idiopathic, heparin-induced thrombocytopenia (HIT) • Loss ↑: blood loss, splenomegaly (e.g. in portal hypertension) • Other causes: gestational trombocytopenia, hereditary thrombocytopenia (e.g. Bernard-Soulier syndrome) • Watch out for pseudothrombocytopenia: false lower result due to agglutination in EDTA tube
White blood cell (WBC) count	• Leukocytes: white blood cells • Part of the immune system	↑ Leukocytosis: • Infections • Inflammatory processes • Autoimmune diseases • Myeloproliferative disease, e.g. leukaemia • Medication-induced, e.g. steroids • Smoking ↓ Leukopenia: • Infections (due to utilisation) • Medication-induced/iatrogenic, e.g. chemotherapy, immunosupressants, antibiotics • Bone marrow deficiency • Splenomegaly (e.g. in portal hypertension) • Benign leukopenia, seen in individuals of African, Middle Eastern, and West Indian descent • Other causes: B12 and folate deficiency

Table 16B // General blood count

LAB VALUE	EXPLANATION	INTERPRETATION
Red blood cell (RBC) count	• Erythrocytes: red blood cells • Transport O_2 and CO_2 between lungs and tissue	↑ Erythrocytosis: • Primary: polycythaemia vera, see Hb • Secondary to oxygen deprivation, see Hb ↓ Erythropenia: • Reduced synthesis: - Nutritional deficiency - Disrupted production in bone marrow • Increased degradation, e.g. autoimmune haemolysis, haemoglobinopathy, DIC, valve haemolysis
Mean corpuscular haemoglobin (MCH)	Average amount of oxygen-carrying haemoglobin per erythrocyte (Hb/erythrocytes)	↑ Hyperchromic anaemia: • Vitamin B12 deficiency • Folic acid deficiency
Mean corpuscular haemoglobin concentration (MCHC)	Average haemoglobin concentration per erythrocyte (Hb/Ht)	= Normochromic anaemia ↓ Hypochromic anaemia: • Iron deficiency • Haemoglobinopathy
Red blood cell distribution width (RDW)	A measure of MCV variance	↑ In case of high MCV variance, e.g. after a blood transfusion or in combined microcytic and macrocytic anaemia (MCV may be normal)
Reticulocyte count (RTIC)	• Reticulocytes: immature erythrocytes that still have RNA • Adequacy of a reticulocyte response depends on haematocrit levels. A deep anaemia should give a marked increase in reticulocyte count.	↑ Reticulocytosis: • Increased erythrocyte synthesis, e.g. haemolytic anaemia, bleeding ↓ Reticulopenia: • Reduced erythrocyte synthesis, e.g. medication-induced myelosuppression, aplastic anaemia, aneamia of chronic disease

Table 16C // General blood count

Anaemia - interpretation

HB	MCV	DIFFERENTIAL DIAGNOSIS
↓	↓	• Iron-deficiency anaemia (chronic blood loss) • Haemoglobinopathy • Other causes: lead poisoning ⊖, sideroblastic anaemia ⊖, hookworm infection ⊖
	↓/=	Anaemia of chronic disease (e.g. infections, malignancy, autoimmune diseases)

Table 17A // Anaemia - interpretation

HB	MCV	DIFFERENTIAL DIAGNOSIS
↓	=	• Acute blood loss • Long-term chronic kidney disease (EPO deficiency) • Malnutrition • Mixed-aetiology anaemias • Multiple myeloma

	=/↑	• Haemolysis
		• Medication-induced
		• Thyroid dysfunction (specifically hypothyroidism)
		• Haematological malignancy
		• Bone marrow disease:
		  - Aplastic anaemia
		  - Bone marrow filtration
		  - Myelodysplastic syndrome

↓	↑	• Vitamin B12 deficiency (e.g. malabsorption, HIV) • Folic acid deficiency • Pregnancy • Toxic: alcohol use disorder, medication-induced (e.g. cytostatics)

Table 17B // Anaemia - interpretation

Arterial blood gas (ABG)

LAB VALUE	EXPLANATION	INTERPRETATION
1. pH 7.35-7.45	Hydrogen ion concentration in the blood	↑ Alkalosis ↓ Acidosis
2. $PaCO_2$ 35-45 mmHg (4.7-6.0 kPa)	Partial pressure of carbon dioxide	↑ • Respiratory acidosis: hypoventilation, type II respiratory insufficiency (e.g. COPD) • Respiratory compensation in metabolic alkalosis ↓ • Respiratory alkalosis: hyperventilation, hyperventilation during hypoxaemia • Respiratory compensation in metabolic acidosis

Table 18A // Arterial blood gas (ABG)

LAB VALUE	EXPLANATION	INTERPRETATION
3. HCO_3^- 22-26 mEQ/L	Buffer for H^+	↑ Metabolic alkalosis: • Loss of H^+: - Gastrointestinal loss (e.g. vomiting, diarrhoea (with Cl^-)) - Renal loss (e.g. activation of RAAS due to primary hyper-aldosteronism, HF, cirrhosis) - Intracellular H^+ shift (as in hypokalaemia) • Increase in HCO_3^-: - Renal retention (e.g. loop and thiazide diuretics) - Cystic fibrosis ↓ Metabolic acidosis: • Increase in H^+: - Excessive production (e.g. ketoacidosis, lactate acidosis, rhabdomyolysis) - Renal insufficiency (impaired H^+ excretion) - Intoxications with exogenous acids (e.g. toxic alcohols, salicylates) - Hyperchloraemia • Loss of HCO_3^-: - Gastrointestinal (e.g. severe diarrhoea, laxative use, gas-trointestinal fistulas) - Renal loss - Medication (e.g. spironolactone)
4. Base excess (BE) -2 to +2 mmol/L	Base excess or deficit needed to get pH to 7.40	↑ • Metabolic alkalosis • Metabolic compensation in respiratory acidosis ↓ • Metabolic acidosis • Metabolic compensation in respiratory alkalosis
5. Anion gap (only in meta-bolic aci-dosis) 4-12 mmol/L	• Number of un-measured an-ions (negatively charged parti-cles, including albumin, SO_4^{2-} and HPO_4^{2-}) • Formula: $[Na^+]$ - $([Cl^-] + [HCO_3^-])$	↑ Due to increase in H^+: • Endogenous: lactic acidosis, ketoacidosis, renal insufficiency • Exogenous: intoxications, e.g. ethylene glycol, methanol, salicylate = Due to loss of HCO_3^- (compensated by higher levels of chloride): • Gastrointestinal loss of HCO_3^- (urine anion gap -) (accompa-nied by Cl^- retention in the kidneys), e.g. diarrhoea • Renal loss (urine anion gap +), e.g. hyperchloraemia • Addison's disease
6. PaO_2 75-100 mmHg 10.0-13.3 kPa	Partial pressure of oxygen	↑ Hyperventilation ↓ Type I respiratory insufficiency: • Hypoventilation • Ventilation perfusion mismatch • Diffusion disorder • Right-to-left shunt

Table 18B // Arterial blood gas (ABG)

LAB VALUE	EXPLANATION	INTERPRETATION
7. SaO_2 ≥95%	Oxygen saturation of haemoglobin	↓ Oxygen deficiency, e.g. pneumonia, carbon monoxide poisoning
8. Lactate 0.5-1.7 mmol/L	End product of anaerobic glycolysis	↑ Diminished tissue oxygenation (lactic acidosis), e.g. sepsis, hypoxaemia

Table 18C // Arterial blood gas (ABG)

- Decreased albumin can result in a false low anion gap (AG) AG = $Na^+ - (Cl^- + HCO_3^-)$.
- Oxygen saturation (SpO_2) measures the saturation of functional Hb = $O_2Hb/(O_2Hb$ + deoxyHb). As a result, the saturation of haemoglobinopathies such as carboxyHb, MetHb, and SulfHb is not measured. In the presence of dyshaemoglobins, oxygen saturation is an unreliable metric (overestimation) and measuring the oxygen fraction is preferred.
- When exposed to 21% oxygen, an air bubble in the sample will cause abnormal pCO_2 (↓) and pO_2 (↑) values due to gas diffusion. With 60% oxygen (e.g. a Venturi mask) → pO_2 will decrease.

Blood gas - interpretation

INTERPRETATION	PH	pCO_2	HCO_3^-	ANION GAP	COMPENSATION MECHANISM
Respiratory alkalosis	↑/=	↓	↓/=		↓ Renal [HCO_3^-] reabsorption (slow)
Metabolic alkalosis	↑/=	↑/=	↑		Hypoventilation (fast)
Respiratory acidosis	↓/=	↑	↑/=		↑ Renal [HCO_3^-] reabsorption (slow)
High anion gap metabolic acidosis	↓/=	↓/=	↓	↑	Hyperventilation
Normal anion gap metabolic acidosis	↓/=	↓/=	↓	=	Hyperventilation

Table 19 // Blood gas - interpretation

The common causes of anion gap acidosis can be recalled using the mnemonic **MUDPILES: m**ethanol, **u**raemia, **d**iabetic ketoacidosis, **p**ropylene glycol, **i**soniazid, **i**ron, **l**actic acidosis, **e**thylene glycol, **s**alicylates.

Electrolytes

Calcium (Ca^{2+}) is partially bound to albumin. Low albumin levels may lead to a decrease in total Ca^{2+} and may be accompanied by normal ionised Ca^{2+}. Total Ca^{2+} can be corrected for the patient's albumin level using lab-specific formulas. Scan the QR code for the formula.

LAB VALUE	EXPLANATION	INTERPRETATION
Sodium (Na^+)	• Main extracellular cation • Very important in water management	↑ Hypernatraemia: • Increased water loss: - Osmotic diarrhoea or diuresis (e.g. hyperglycaemia, mannitol) - Arginine vasopressin deficiency (e.g. cranial trauma, infections, autoimmune) - Arginine vasopressin resistance (e.g. drugs, amyloidosis, hereditary) • Increased sodium retention (iatrogenic with unchecked IV drip) • Insufficient fluid intake (with or without intact thirst stimulus) ↓ Hyponatraemia: often multiple causes • Water retention: - Syndrome of inappropriate antidiuretic hormone secretion (SIADH) - Renal insufficiency stage 5 - Congestive HF - Liver cirrhosis - Blood loss (resulting in ADH ↑ to preserve volume) - Nephrotic syndrome • Increased sodium loss: - Gastrointestinal, e.g. diarrhoea, small bowel obstruction - Renal, e.g. diuretics, renal failure, osmotic diuresis (severe hyperglycaemia), Addison's disease - Transdermal, e.g. burns, excessive sweating • Other: - Tea & toast (malnutrition) - Polydipsia

Table 20A // Electrolytes

LAB VALUE	EXPLANATION	INTERPRETATION
Potassium (K^+)	• Main intracellular cation • Regulates e.g. nerve impulse transmission, glycogen and protein synthesis	↑ Hyperkalaemia: • Extracellular redistribution (shift): - Metabolic or respiratory acidosis - Hyperosmolality - Insulin deficiency - Medication-induced, e.g. beta blockers, digoxin • Tissue breakdown (often in combination with LDH, AST, bilirubin): - Haemolysis - Tumorlysis - Rhabdomyolysis - Distal arterial occlusion • Impaired renal excretion: - Mineralocorticoid deficiency - Renal insufficiency - Medication-induced, e.g. ACE inhibitors, NSAIDs, potassium-sparing diuretics - Type IV renal tubular acidosis • Pseudohyperkalaemia (e.g. following blood collection) ↓ Hypokalaemia: • Intracellular redistribution: - Metabolic or respiratory alkalosis - Insulin use • Renal loss: - Renal conditions, e.g. type I and II renal tubular acidosis - Hyperaldosteronism - Medication-induced, e.g. diuretics, glucocorticoids - Hypomagnesaemia - Chronic metabolic acidosis • Extrarenal loss, e.g. gastrointestinal (diarrhoea) • Insufficient intake, e.g. chronic alcohol use disorder

Table 20B // Electrolytes

ACE, Angiotensin-converting enzyme; ADH, antidiuretic hormone; AST, Aspartate aminotransferase; IV, intravenous; LDH, Lactate dehydrogenase; NSAID, non-steroidal anti-inflammatory drugs; PPI, proton pump inhibitor; PTH, parathyroid hormone; SIADH, Syndrome of inappropriate antidiuretic hormone ADH release; TPN, total parenteral nutrition

LAB VALUE	EXPLANATION	INTERPRETATION
Magnesium (Mg^{2+})	• 70% in bone, remainder is intracellular • Cofactor in enzymatic processes • Stabilises nucleic acids and ribosomes	↑ Hypermagnesaemia: • Renal insufficiency • Medication-induced, e.g. laxatives, lithium, antacids containing magnesium • Other: - Rhabdomyolysis - Hypothyroidism ↓ Hypomagnesaemia: • Gastrointestinal loss, e.g. diarrhoea, inadequate intake, malnutrition/malabsorption • Medication-induced, e.g. PPIs, diuretics, cisplatina, insulin, tacrolimus, cyclosporine • Renal loss, e.g. hyperaldosteronism, hyperthyroidism, diuretics • Other: - Chronic alcohol use - Hypercalcaemia - Hungry bone syndrome
Chloride (Cl^-)	• Main extracellular anion • Regulation closely linked to sodium metabolism	↑ Hyperchloraemia: • Chloride administration: secondary to administration of chloride-rich IV fluids • True water loss relative to chloride: - Renal: osmotic diuresis, postobstructive diuresis, arginine vasopressine resistance (formerly diabetes insipidus) - Extrarenal: fever, diarrhoea, burns, dehydration • Increase in tubular reabsorption: e.g. renal tubular acidosis, acetazolamide, neobladder ↓ Hypochloraemia: • Increased loss: - Gastrointestinal, e.g. vomiting - Renal - Ascites - True water gain relative to chloride: congestive HF, syndrome of inappropriate antidiuretic hormone secretion (SIADH) - High output stoma • Metabolic alkalosis

Table 20C // Electrolytes

LAB VALUE	EXPLANATION	INTERPRETATION
Calcium (Ca^{2+})	• 99% is stored in bone as a mineral, 50% of plasma calcium is free and biologically active (ionised), 40% is bound to albumin, 10% bound to organic molecules • Regulates e.g. nerve impulse conduction, muscle contractility, enzyme functioning, and clotting	↑ Hypercalcaemia: • Primary/tertiary hyperparathyroidism • Tumour-induced, e.g. bone metastases, multiple myeloma, PTH-like peptide • Endocrine: hyperthyroidism, adrenal cortex insufficiency, pheochromocytoma • Vitamin D excessive production or intoxication (e.g. sarcoidosis, lymphoma) • Pseudohypercalcaemia ↓ Hypocalcaemia: • Primary hypoparathyroidism • PTH resistance/pseudohypoparathyroidism • Vitamin D deficiency • Chronic renal insufficiency • Hypomagnesaemia • Medication-induced, e.g. corticosteroids, diuretics, anti-seizure medication • Malabsorption • Acute pancreatitis • Blood transfusions, including massive blood transfusions
Phosphate (PO_4^{3-})	• 75% in bone, remainder in muscle tissue and intracellularly • Main intracellular anion • Particularly important for cell energy metabolism	↑ Hyperphosphataemia: • Endogenous: rhabdomyolysis, haemolysis, intestinal infarction • Exogenous: supplementation, e.g. phosphate enemas • Reduced renal excretion: acute or chronic renal insufficiency, hypoparathyroidism, medication-induced (e.g. vitamin D supplementation) • Shift from intracellular: lactate acidosis, ketoacidosis • Pseudohyperphosphataemia: hyperbilirubinaemia, extreme hypertriglyceridaemia, heparin ↓ Hypophosphataemia: • Redistribution: refeeding syndrome, respiratory alkalosis, diabetic ketoacidosis, hungry bone syndrome, medication-induced (e.g. insulin) • Renal loss: hyperparathyroidism, vitamin D deficiency, medication-induced (e.g. diuretics, glucocorticoids) • Reduced absorption: TPN, malabsorption, anorexia nervosa, alcohol use disorder, chronic/non-chronic diarrhoea, vitamin D deficiency, medication-induced (e.g. overuse of antacids)
Bicarbonate (HCO_3^-)		See Arterial blood gas

Table 20D // Electrolytes

Liver tests and pancreatic tests

LAB VALUE	EXPLANATION	INTERPRETATION
Alanine transaminase (ALT)	Enzyme found primarily in hepatocytes	↑ • Liver conditions: - Hepatitis, e.g. viral, toxic, alcoholic (ALT<AST), autoimmune, ischaemic - Non-alcoholic steatohepatitis - Liver cirrhosis - Hepatocellular carcinoma/liver metastases - Medication-induced liver injury - Liver abscess - Acute liver failure - Haemochromatosis - Wilson's disease - Primary biliary cholangitis/primary sclerosing cholangitis • Bile duct obstruction, see ALP • Chronic/acute pancreatitis • Budd-Chiari syndrome • Preeclampsia/eclampsia/HELLP • Hypotension, i.e. septic shock
Aspartate aminotransferase (AST)	Enzyme found mainly in liver and striated (i.e. cardiac, skeletal) muscle tissue	↑ • In all diagnoses mentioned in ALT • May also be elevated in: - Myocardial infarction/HF - Muscle conditions, e.g. rhabdomyolysis, dermatomyositis
Alkaline phosphatase (ALP)	Enzyme found primarily in liver parenchyma, bile epithelium, and osteoblasts	↑ • Bile duct obstruction: - Cholelithiasis - Cholangitis - Hepatocellular carcinoma, cholangiocarcinoma, liver metastases - Pancreatic malignancy - Medication-induced - Pregnancy • Liver conditions: - Hepatitis, e.g. alcoholic - Primary biliary cholangitis - Primary sclerosing cholangitis • Bone disease (isolated elevation of ALP): - Hyperparathyroidism - Bone metastases - Paget's disease - Osteomyelitis or fractures

Table 21A // Liver tests and pancreatic tests

<table>
<tr><th>LAB VALUE</th><th>EXPLANATION</th><th>INTERPRETATION</th></tr>
<tr><td>Gamma-glutamyl-transferase (GGT)</td><td>• Enzyme present in virtually all cells
• Serum GGT generally comes from the hepatobiliary system</td><td>↑ • Bile duct obstruction, see ALP
• Liver conditions:
- Primary biliary cholangitis
- Primary sclerosing cholangitis
- Hepatitis, e.g. alcoholic
• Alcohol use
• Obesity</td></tr>
<tr><td>Bilirubin</td><td>• Degradation product of haemoglobin
• Mainly formed in the spleen → conjugated in the liver → excreted with bile</td><td>↑ Hyperbilirubinaemia:
• Pre-hepatic (unconjugated): excessive formation of bilirubin (direct bilirubin <20%), e.g. haemolysis, haematoma resorption
• Hepatic (unconjugated and conjugated): liver disease, Gilbert's disease
• Post-hepatic (conjugated): bile duct obstruction (direct bilirubin >50%, ALP ↑, GGT ↑)</td></tr>
<tr><td>Lactate dehydrogenase (LDH)</td><td>Enzyme involved in glycolysis in various tissues</td><td>↑ • Increased cellular death in:
- Liver conditions
- Myocardial infarction
- Muscle conditions
- Haemolysis
• Malignancies (specifically lymphoma, haematological malignancy)</td></tr>
<tr><td>Lipase</td><td>• Enzyme that hydrolyses triglycerides to fatty acids and glycerides
• Serum lipase is largely pancreas-specific
• Released into circulation during autolysis of pancreatic tissue
• Lipase has a higher sensitivity for pancreatitis and is released more often than amylase</td><td>↑ • Acute pancreatitis (with acute or chronic pancreatitis there might be no elevation)
• May also be elevated in:
- Renal insufficiency
- DKA
- Bile duct disease
↓ Exocrine pancreatic insufficiency</td></tr>
<tr><td>Amylase</td><td>• Enzyme produced in the pancreas and salivary glands
• Involved in polysaccharide degradation</td><td>↑ • Acute pancreatitis
• May also be elevated in:
- Salivary gland disorders
- Renal insufficiency
- Intra-abdominal inflammation
- Bile duct disease
↓ Exocrine pancreatic insufficiency</td></tr>
</table>

Table 21B // Liver tests and pancreatic tests

A combination of elevated AST and ALT (liver enzymes) indicates hepatocellular damage. The AST/ALT ratio can provide information about the underlying condition. ALT>AST could indicate viral or autoimmune hepatitis and AST>ALT could indicate alcoholic hepatitis. A combination of bilirubin ↑, ALP ↑, and GGT ↑ indicates cholestasis.

A decrease in the synthetic function of the liver indicates severe liver disease. The common tests for assessing liver synthetic function are albumin, PT/INT, and glucose.

Inflammatory markers

LAB VALUE	EXPLANATION	INTERPRETATION
Erythrocyte sedimentation rate (ESR)	• Erythrocyte sedimentation rate (mm/h) • Elevated with increased concentration of acute-phase proteins and/or immunoglobulin-mediated surface charge alteration, causing erythrocytes to repel each other less and sink faster	↑ • Increased blood protein levels: - Infections - Autoimmune diseases - Rheumatic conditions - Malignancies - Monoclonal and polyclonal gammopathies - Infarction - Hypothyroidism • Anaemia • Pregnancy, obesity, older age, smoking ↓ • Abnormalities of erythrocytes, e.g. polycythaemia, sickle cell disease • Congestive HF • Hypogammaglobulinaemia
C-reactive protein (CRP)	• C-reactive protein • Positive acute-phase protein • Produced in the liver	↑ • Infections • Inflammation • Rheumatic conditions • Malignancies • Trauma • Thrombosis

Table 22A // Inflammatory markers

In various inflammations, e.g. in acute pancreatitis an elevated WBC precedes an increase in CRP (approx. 24h).

LAB VALUE	EXPLANATION	INTERPRETATION
Leukocyte differential	Breakdown of total leukocytes by subtype	↑ Neutrophilia: • Bacterial infection, sepsis, myeloproliferative diseases ↓ Neutropenia: • Decreased production: severe infections, medication-induced/iatrogenic • Increased utilisation/destruction: medication-induced antibody formation ↑ Lymphocytosis: • Infection, smoking, hyposplenism, lymphoproliferative disease ↓ Lymphopenia: • Infection, HIV, renal failure ↑ Monocytosis: • Bacterial/parasitic infection, myeloproliferative diseases, Hodgkin's disease, neutropenia, steroids ↓ Monopenia: • In neutropenia, hairy cell leukaemia, cytotoxic agents (e.g. chemotherapy) ↑ Eosinophilia: • Parasitic infection, allergic reactions, skin diseases, myeloproliferative diseases, hypereosinophilic syndrome ↑ Basophilia: • Allergic reactions, iron deficiency, chronic myeloid leukaemia, systemic mastocytosis, allergic reaction

Table 22B // Inflammatory markers

Renal function tests

LAB VALUE	EXPLANATION	INTERPRETATION
Creatinine	Degradation product of creatinine phosphate from muscle tissue, mainly excreted by glomerular filtration	↑ • Acute kidney injury, chronic kidney disease • Medication-induced, e.g. trimethoprim, supplements • Dehydration • Muscle breakdown (e.g. rhabdomyolysis, myocardial infarction) • Excessive meat consumption ↓ • Significant fluid overload • Low protein intake, e.g. malnutrition • Reduced muscle mass, e.g. increasing age, females • Hyperthyroidism

Table 23A // Renal function tests
CKD-EPI, Chronic Kidney Disease Epidemiology Collaboration

LAB VALUE	EXPLANATION	INTERPRETATION
Creatinine-clearance	Plasma (in ml) cleared of creatinine per minute by glomerular filtration and secretion. Both serum creatinine and urine creatinine (24h collection) levels are needed.	• Prerenal kidney disease (decreased renal perfusion): e.g. hypovolaemia, hypotension, decreased circulating volume (e.g. congestive HF, hepatorenal syndrome), renal artery stenosis, medication-induced • Renal kidney disease (reduced clearance due to impaired glomeruli and/or tubules): e.g. acute tubular necrosis (e.g. ischaemia, nephrotoxic drugs), interstitial nephritis, DM, medication-induced • Postrenal kidney disease (urinary tract obstruction): e.g. urolithiasis, prostate carcinoma, benign prostatic hyperplasia, urinary retention
Estimated glomerular filtration rate (eGFR, CKD-EPI)	• Estimation of GFR based on serum creatinine, sex, age, ethnicity, and weight as a marker for muscle mass • Relevant in chronic kidney disease (stages 1-5) • Only reliable in more or less stable kidney function	
Osmolality	• Number of particles dissolved in 1 kg serum (osmolarity: in 1L) • Formula for 'effective osmolality': 2 × [Na^+] + [glucose]	↑ Increased level of osmoles, e.g. Na^+, glucose, urea, or exogenous osmoles, e.g. toxic alcohols ↓ Decreased level of osmoles, e.g. Na^+, glucose, urea
Osmol gap	• Measured osmolality – calculated osmolality • A high osmol gap (>10-20 mOsm/kg) is defined as the measured osmolality minus 2 x [Na^+] + [glucose] + [urea]	↑ Increased Na^+, glucose, urea, or other osmotically active substances, e.g. toxic alcohols, ketone bodies
Urea	• Waste product of hepatic protein metabolism • Reabsorbed in the kidneys	↑ • Prerenal, renal, or postrenal kidney disease (if urea/creatinine ratio ↑: prerenal) • Dehydration • Increased protein degradation, e.g. tissue damage, upper gastrointestinal bleeding • High-protein diet ↓ • Haemodilution • Pregnancy • Malabsorption/malnutrition • Severe liver damage

Table 23B // Renal function tests

LAB VALUE	EXPLANATION	INTERPRETATION
Uric acid/urate	End product of purine metabolism	↑ • Increased production: - Genetic - Idiopathic - Increased tissue breakdown, e.g. infections, malignancies - Increased nucleic acid metabolism, e.g. leukaemia, lymphoma, haemolytic anaemia • Reduced renal secretion, e.g. renal insufficiency ↓ • Xanthine oxidase deficiency • Medication-induced
Fractional excretion of sodium	Percentage of the glomerular filtered sodium that is eventually excreted in the urine	↑ • In AKI: indicates intrarenal aetiology • In hypotonic hyponatremia: indicated renal cause ↓ • In AKI: indicated a prerenal cause • In hypotonic hyponatremia: indicates extrarenal cause

Table 23C // Renal function tests

Acute kidney disease - interpretation

ACUTE KIDNEY DISEASE	PRE-RENAL	RENAL
Osmolality (urine)	>500 mOsmol/kg	<350 mOsmol/kg
Na^+ (urine)	<20 mmol/L	>40 mmol/L
Urea/creatinine ratio (serum)	>0.1 mmol/μmol	<0.1 mmol/μmol

Table 24 // Acute kidney disease - interpretation

The 'effective osmolality' is important because these osmotically active substances cannot pass the semi-permanent cell membrane, and thus can cause water shifts (such as cerebral oedema). Urea, for example, can pass freely through the cell membrane and is unlikely to cause water shifts.

Clotting markers

LAB VALUE	EXPLANATION	INTERPRETATION
International normalised ratio (INR)	• Calculation based on prothrombin time (PT) • Measure of the extrinsic and common pathway of the coagulation cascade • Monitoring vitamin K antagonists • Patient plasma PT/ normalised plasma PT	↑ • If prolonged PT + normal aPTT: - Use of vitamin K antagonists (coumarines or warfarin) - Isolated factor VII deficiency - Coagulation disorders, e.g. coagulopathy or mild vitamin K deficiency - In acute or chronic liver failure. If chronic → progression of advanced liver cirrhosis. - Acute DIC • If prolonged PT + prolonged aPTT: - Factor I, II, V, X, or fibrinogen deficiency, combined factor deficiencies - Liver failure - Acute DIC - Severe vitamin K deficiency - Anticoagulants (e.g. warfarin, direct thrombin inhibitors, others) ↓ Activation of clotting in early DIC
Prothrombin test/ time (PT)	Test for the extrinsic and common pathway of the coagulation cascade	
Activated partial thromboplastin test/time (aPTT)	• Test for the intrinsic and common pathway of the coagulation cascade • Monitoring unfractionated heparin therapy	↑ If prolonged aPTT + normal PT: • Factor VIII (haemophilia A), factor IX (haemophilia B), factor XI (haemophilia C) deficiency • Factor XII deficiency • Von Willebrand disease • Anticoagulants (unfractionated heparin therapy) • Lupus anticoagulant ↓ • Strong elevation one or more clotting factors (e.g. factor VIII due to stress) • Activation of coagulation in early DIC • Pregnancy (factor VIII ↑ and fibrinogen ↑)
D-dimer	Degradation product of fibrinolysis	↑ • Venous thrombosis (high sensitivity but low specificity) • Pulmonary embolism (high sensitivity but low specificity) • DIC • Other causes (low specificity): - Pregnancy - Infection - Renal insufficiency - Trauma - Malignancies - Aortic dissection

Table 25A // Clotting markers
t-PA, tissue plasminogen activator

LAB VALUE	EXPLANATION	INTERPRETATION
Fibrino-gen	• Coagulation factor produced in the liver • Converted into fibrin by thrombin • Positive acute-phase protein	↑ • Inflammatory processes • Trauma • Pregnancy ↓ • Decreased synthesis, e.g. liver disease • Increased degradation: - DIC - Fibrinolysis • Increased loss, e.g. after bleeding • Medication-induced, e.g. t-PA, streptokinase

Table 25B // Clotting markers

Coumarin derivative therapy can be monitored by tracking INR, heparin therapy by tracking aPTT, and LMWH therapy by tracking anti-Xa activity. Monitoring of therapy with DOACs is employed in specific cases, e.g. when using DOACs in patients with a gastric bypass. Therapy with platelet aggregation inhibitors is not monitored in practice.

Laboratories use different techniques to measure prothrombin time (PT), which makes PT values very difficult to compare. The INR is therefore used to correct for differences between labs.

Miscellaneous

LAB VALUE	EXPLANATION	INTERPRETATION
Ammo-nia	Degradation product of proteolysis	↑ Hyperammonaemia: • Congenital urea cycle enzyme defects • Acquired: - Liver cirrhosis (90%) - Infections - Multiple myeloma - Acute leukaemia - Medication-induced

Table 26A // Miscellaneous
IM, intramuscular

LAB VALUE	EXPLANATION	INTERPRETATION
Glucose	• Blood sugar • Main energy source for all cellular processes	↑ Hyperglycaemia: • Impaired glucose tolerance, DM, diabetes gravidarum • Acute stress: trauma, sepsis, myocardial infarction, cerebrovascular accident • Medication: corticosteroids • Endocrinopathy: Cushing's syndrome, acromegaly ↓ Hypoglycaemia: • Medication-induced, e.g. sulphonylurea derivatives, insulin • Insulinoma • Fasting/malnutrition, alcohol • Liver failure • Endocrinopathy: hypocortisolism, panhypopituitarism
Creatine kinase (CK)	• Enzyme needed for e.g. muscle contraction • Predominantly found in skeletal muscle, brain, and heart • Has various isoenzymes	↑ Increased cellular death in: • Muscle conditions: myositis, rhabdomyolysis, overtraining, intramuscular (IM) injection, hereditary muscle diseases, malignant hypertension • Myocardial infarction (often used to estimate infarction size) • Epilepsy • Hypothyroidism • Trauma/postoperative
Lactate	• End product of anaerobic glycolysis • Produced by muscle cells and red blood cells, especially in hypoxic state	↑ • Hypoxic states • Dehydration • Shock • Severe anaemia • Severe liver/kidney disease • Medication-induced (e.g. metformin, propofol), toxic (e.g. methanol, carbon monoxide)

Table 26B // Miscellaneous

Cardiac markers

LAB VALUE	EXPLANATION	INTERPRETATION
(NT-pro)BNP BNP <100 ng/L NT-proBNP <125 ng/L	• BNP and the physiologically inactive cleavage product NT-proBNP • Produced in the heart in response to increased pressure and ventricular stretching • Active natriuretic • Used to rule out congestive HF	↑ • Congestive HF • Other possible causes: - Renal insufficiency - Pulmonary embolism - Pulmonary oedema - Atrial fibrillation - Sepsis, liver cirrhosis, hyperthyroidism - Structural or congenital heart disease ↓ • Obesity • Female sex

Table 27A // Cardiac markers

LAB VALUE	EXPLANATION	INTERPRETATION
Troponins TnI/ TnT	• Myocardial proteins involved in muscle contraction and relaxation • Used to detect/rule out myocardial cell damage due to acute myocardial infarction	↑ • Acute myocardial infarction • May also be elevated in: - Type II myocardial ischaemia - Non-ischaemic myocardial damage, e.g. myocarditis, sepsis, myocardial injury (e.g. contusion cordis) - Renal insufficiency (troponin T) - Pulmonary embolism

Table 27B // Cardiac markers

ECG

The electrocardiogram (ECG) is one of the most commonly used examinations in acute medicine and has numerous indications: including chest pains, palpitations, dyspnoea, syncope, (suspected) electrolyte imbalances and intoxications. In this section, we will discuss the basic principles of electrocardiography and the systematic evaluation of the ECG. See section *The treatment of a patient with...* for specific applications of the ECG and the section *Conditions* for context-specific ECG characteristics.

Basic principles of the ECG

An ECG is a safe, non-invasive test in which electrodes are used to measure the electrical activity of the heart. It is important to interpret ECGs systematically. Indications for an ECG include palpitations, dyspnoea, chest pain (CP), epigastric pain, intoxication, cyanosis, syncope, reduced exercise tolerance, monitoring of critically ill patients, electrolyte disturbances, follow-up of hypertension, diabetes mellitus (DM) and heart disease. Allergy for ECG electrodes is a relative contraindication for an ECG. In these cases hypoallergenic electrodes can be used.

A standard ECG consists of 12 leads, including six limb leads that visualise the frontal plane (I, II, III, aVR, aVL, aVF) and six precordial leads that visualise the axial plane (V1-V6), see Figure 10. See Table 28 for the location of precordial ECG electrodes. The leads pick up electrical activity moving towards a particular part of the heart and project it as a deflection on the ECG. See Table 29 for an overview of the leads and the corresponding areas of the heart. Electrical cardiac activity moving towards the positive electrode is shown as a positive deflection on the ECG, while electrical activity moving away from the positive electrode is projected as a negative deflection.

ECGs are printed on ECG paper (see Figure 10). The horizontal axis shows the time, with each large square representing 0.2 sec and each small square representing 0.04 sec (at a standard paper speed of 25 mm/sec). The vertical axis shows the voltage, with each small square representing 0.1 mV and each large square representing 0.5 mV (with standard 10 mm/mV calibration).

LEAD	POSITION
V1	4th intercostal space (ICS) parasternal right
V2	4th ICS parasternal left
V3	Between V2 and V4
V4	5th ICS midclavicular left
V5	Anterior axillary line on the left at the same horizontal level as V4
V6	Midaxillary left at the same horizontal level as V4

Table 28 // Positioning of the ECG electrodes

LEAD	PART OF THE HEART
II, III, AVF	Inferior
V1, V2	Anteroseptal
V3, V4	Anterior
I, AVL, V5, V6	Lateral

Table 29 // Positioning of the ECG leads

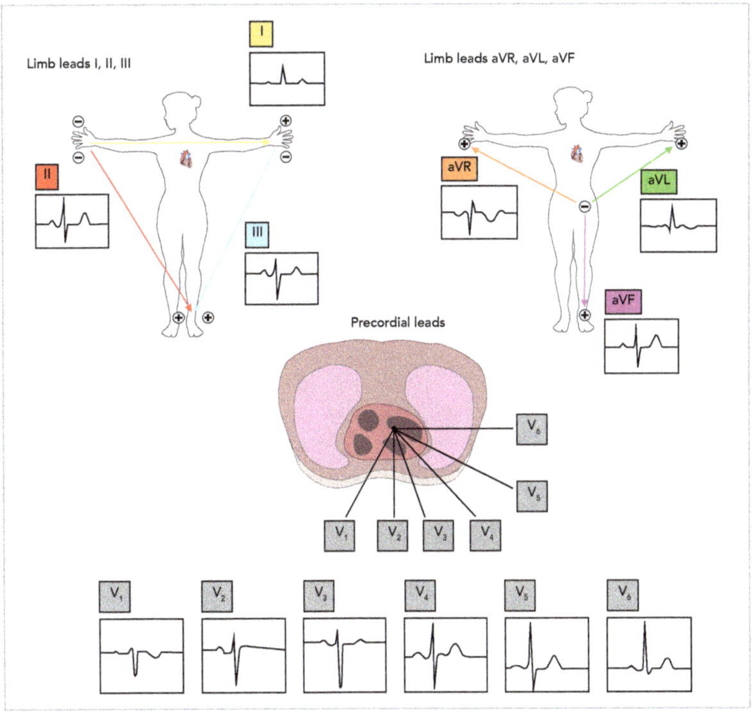

Figure 10 // ECG leads

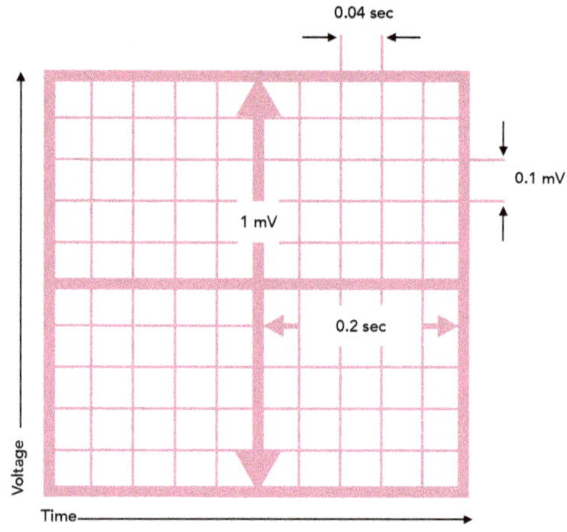

Figure 11 // Standard ECG paper

An ECG can be used to distinguish several components and details of the cardiac cycle (see Figure 12). With a sinus rhythm, an impulse is generated in the sinus node, leading to the depolarisation of the atria, which is represented by the P wave on ECG. This is followed by an isoelectric segment called the PR interval or PTa segment, which reflects the conduction of the impulse through the AV node.

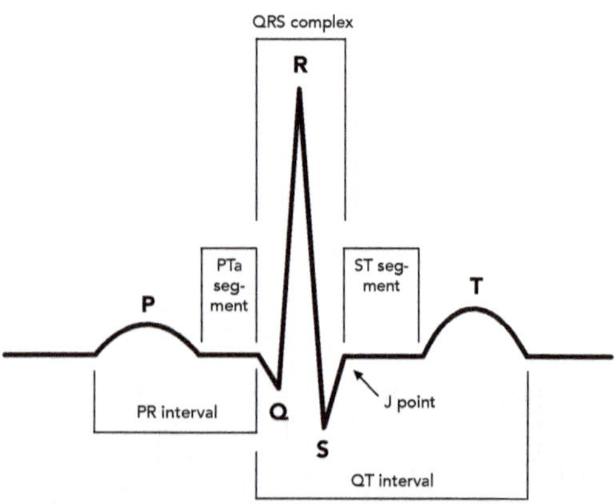

Figure 12 // ECG components

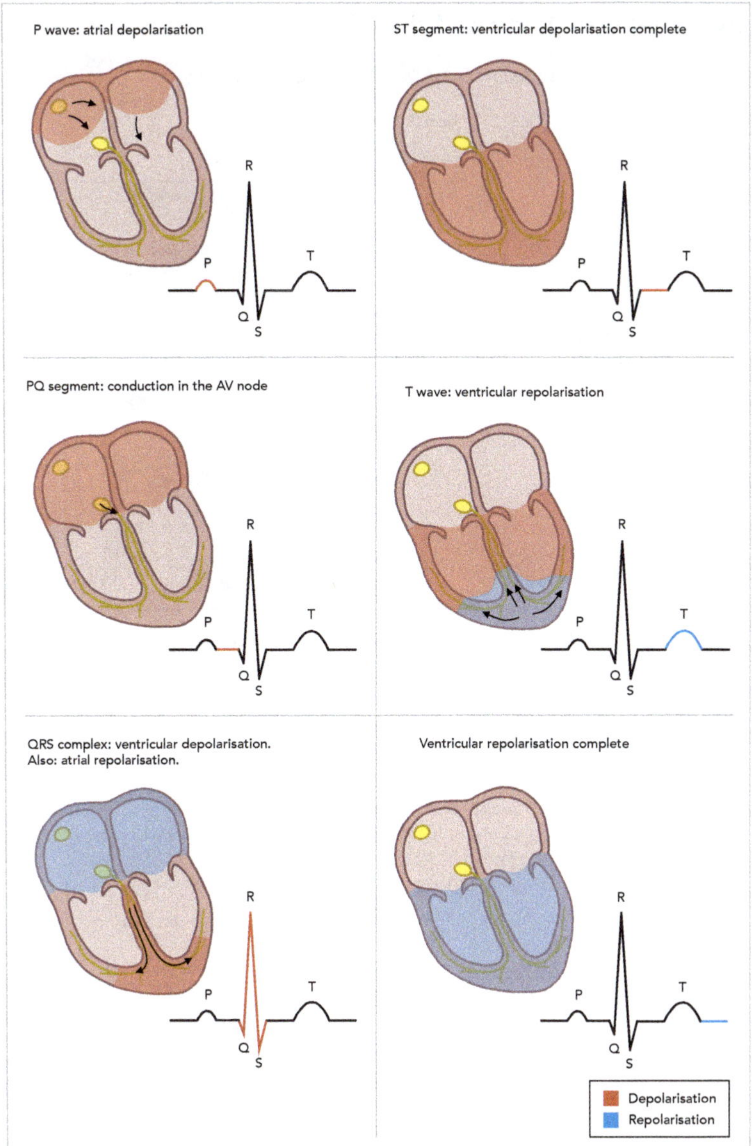

Figure 13 // Physiology of ECG components

Systematic evaluation of the ECG

PERSONAL DATA & TECHNICAL QUALITY	
Check personal data	

Check calibration and paper speed (for an example of standard ECG paper, see Figure 11)

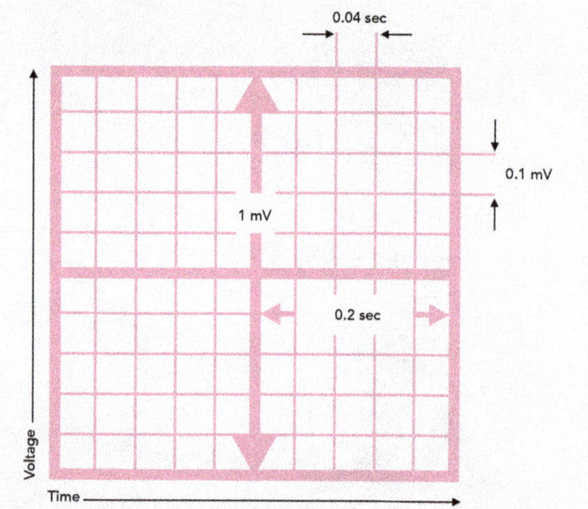

Check placement and orientation of ECG leads	
Left arm/right arm reversal	Negative complex in I with negative P wave. Most common cause of right heart axis.
Neutral lead placed on arm instead of leg	Lead I, II or III (depending on the reversal) measures the potential difference between the two legs. Because this difference is negligible, the lead will show a flatline, with the possible exception of some far-field potential (i.e. electrical activity of the heart occurring far away from the lead, visualised as minuscule deflections on ECG). If the neutral lead is misplaced, almost all other leads will look abnormal too.
Chest lead reversals	Unexpected R-wave progression (e.g. increase - decrease - increase)

Table 30 // Personal data and technical quality

Incorrect placement of ECG leads can lead to inversion of limb leads of microvoltages in the chest leads.

RHYTHM	
In a sinus rhythm, each P wave must be followed by a QRS complex and each QRS complex must be preceded by a P wave. The P wave must also be sinusoidal, which means it must be biphasic in V1 and positive in II and aVF. The positive deflections in II and aVF are caused by the direction of atrial activation (down from the sinus node, i.e. towards II and aVF). In an atrial rhythm, the atrium is activated from a focus other than the sinus node, which results in a different shape depending on the origin of the impulse.	
Sinus rhythm	P wave is positive in I, II; biphasic in V1
Atrial flutter	Sawtooth wave on baseline, often regular, 300/min with 2:1 AV block
Atrial fibrillation	Irregular, no uniform P waves
Atrial rhythm	Abnormal P wave before each QRS complex
Junctional/ventricular escape rhythm	No P wave before each QRS complex

Table 31 // Rhythm

RATE	
Normal	60-100/min
Bradycardia	<60/min
Tachycardia	>100/min
Narrow complex tachycardia	→ always supraventricular
Wide complex tachycardia	→ ventricular or supraventricular tachycardia with bundle branch block (or aberrancy)
Regular rate: count number of large squares between R waves: 300-150-100-75-60-50 Irregular rate: count number of QRS complexes in 30 large squares (6 sec) x 10	

Table 32 // Rates

CONDUCTION TIMES	
PQ interval	**120-200 ms**
First-degree AV block	PQ >200 ms
Second-degree type I/ Wenckebach AV block	Gradually increasing PQ interval until impulses from the atria are no longer conducted to the ventricles.

Table 33A // Conduction times

CONDUCTION TIMES	
PQ interval	**120-200 ms**
Second-degree type II/ Mobitz II AV block	Sudden failure of impulse conduction from the atria to the ventricles (P wave not followed by QRS complex). PQ interval need not be prolonged.
Third-degree AV block	No impulse conduction from the atria to the ventricles (AV dissociation: independent P waves and QRS complexes on ECG). Atria and ventricles contract completely independently, both at their own constant rate. Frequently results in an escape rhythm of 50/min.
QRS complex	**80-120 ms**
Left bundle branch block (LBBB)	• QRS >120 ms • Negative in V1 • Wide R, no Q in I, aVL, V5, V6 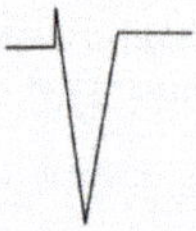 LBBB
Incomplete LBBB	QRS 100-120 ms, LBBB characteristics
Right bundle branch block (RBBB)	• QRS >120 ms • Positive in V1 • RSR' in V1 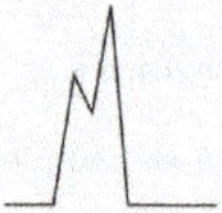 RBBB
Incomplete RBBB	QRS 100-120 ms, RBBB characteristics
Delayed intraventricular conduction	QRS >120 ms and no typical LBBB or RBBB characteristics
QTc	**♂ <450 ms, ♀ <460 ms**

- The QT interval is measured from the onset of the QRS complex to the end of the T wave (see Figure 11).
- The duration of the QT interval is linked to the heart rate: the faster the heart beats, the shorter the QT interval. The QT interval should always be corrected for heart rate, resulting in the corrected QT interval or QTc.
- Measure the QT interval in the lead where the QT interval is longest.
- General rule: the QT interval is probably normal if QT <50% of the RR interval.

Table 33B // Conduction times

CARDIAC AXIS

The electrical cardiac axis is a vector that reflects the average direction of the overall electrical activity of the ventricle, and can be determined with the limb leads. A normal cardiac axis is between -30° and +90°. The cardiac axis is determined by assessing whether the QRS complex is positive (+) or negative (-) in leads I, II and aVF.

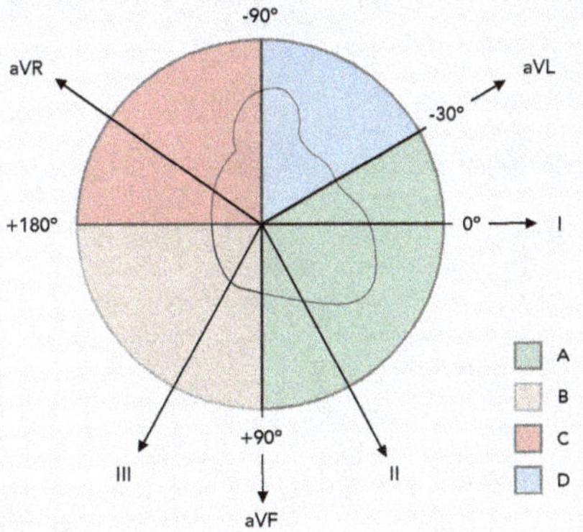

A. Normal/intermediate cardiac axis

B. Right cardiac axis

- Physiological (children, adolescents)
- Right ventricular hypertrophy
- Left posterior hemiblock

C. Extreme cardiac axis

- Always indicates pathology
- Always check that the electrodes are positioned correctly

D. Left cardiac axis

- Inferior infarction
- Left anterior hemiblock

Table 34 // Cardiac axis

P WAVE & PR SEGMENT

Normal P wave	• Positive in I and II • Biphasic in V1 • Monomorphic
Left atrial enlargement	• Terminal negative portion in V1 >1 mm^2 • P wave > 40 ms in II
Right atrial enlargement	• P >2.5 mm in II, III, aVF or • P >1.5 mm in V1

Table 35 // P wave & PR segment

QRS COMPLEX

Pathological Q wave	• Every Q in V1-V3 • Q width >30 ms in I, II, III, aVL, aVF, V4-V6 • Q depth >1 mm • In at least two adjacent leads
Left ventricular hypertrophy (LVH)	• R in V5/V6 + S in V1 >35 mm (Sokolow) • R aVL + S V3 >28 mm ♂ / >20 mm ♀ (Cornell) • R aVL >12 mm (Lewis)

Table 36A // QRS complex

QRS COMPLEX	
Microvoltages	• QRS <5 mm in all limb leads • QRS <10 mm in all precordial leads
R-wave progression	• R-wave amplitude increases in V1-V5 • R wave > S deflection in V3-V6

Table 36B // QRS complex

ST SEGMENT	
Measure	J-point elevation above baseline (see Figure 12)
Significant ST elevation	New ST elevation at the J-point in at least two contiguous leads: • ≥2.5 mm in ♂ <40y, ≥2 mm in ♂ ≥40y, or ≥1.5 mm in ♀ regardless of age in leads V2–V3 • and/or ≥1 mm in the other leads (in the absence of left ventricular hypertrophy or LBBB)
Localising infarctions using involved leads	• II, III, aVF: inferior • V1, V2: anteroseptal • V3, V4: anterior • I, aVL, V5, V6: lateral

Table 37 // ST segment

T WAVE	
Negative T wave	Normal in aVR, V1, III, with negative QRS complex
Pathological T wave	• Flat: T <0.5 mm in I, II, V3-V6 • Negative: T >-0.5 mm in I, II, V3-V6
Enlarged T wave	• Hyperacute ischemia • Hyperkalaemia

Table 38 // T top

COMPARE WITH AN OLD ECG IF AVAILABLE
Deliberately watch for new LBBB, pathological Qs, ST segment abnormalities, axis deviations and poor R-wave progression

Table 39 // Compare with old ECG

CONCLUSION
Take a brief note of your findings with regard to rhythm, rate, conduction times, cardiac axis and the individual components of the cardiac cycle. End with an overarching conclusion.

Table 40 // Conclusion

$$QTc = \frac{QT}{\sqrt{RR\text{ - interval (sec)}}}$$

Formula 1 // QTc calculation with Bazett's formula

Imaging

See the pocket *Radiology* for more information about radiological imaging techniques, indications, and interpretation.

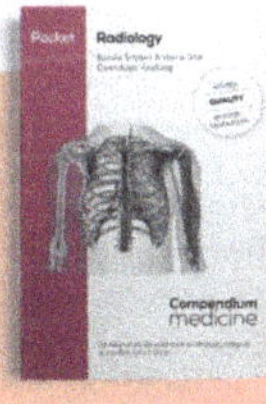

Conventional X-ray

A conventional X-ray, or radiograph, uses X-rays (photons) to create radiological images. X-rays can be partially absorbed (i.e. dense structures, such as bone or metal) or pass through (i.e. hypodense structures, such as air or fat).

EXAM	INDICATIONS	ASSESSMENT
Chest X-ray	• Trauma (e.g. fractures, lung contusion, pneumothorax, hemothorax) • Infection (e.g. pneumonia, mediastinal emphysema, TB (tuberculosis)) • Other airway pathology (e.g. atelectasis, bronchopathy) • Screening for vascular pathology (e.g. aortic aneurysm, congenital vascular disease) • Screening for tumours (primary lung tumour, metastases, lymphadenopathy, pleural fluid) • Cardiac pathology (e.g. cardiomegaly, tamponade, fluid overload) • Lines (e.g. central venous lines, portacath, tube, pacemakers/ICD, nasogastric tube)	Systematic chest X-ray assessment using **ABCDEF**: • **A**ssessment of technical quality, **A**irways • **B**ones and soft tissue • **C**ardiac and mediastinal silhouette • **D**iaphragm and gastric bubble • **E**ffusions (pleural) • **F**ields of the lungs

Table 41 // Chest X-ray indications and assessment

EXAM	INDICATIONS	CASE IMAGES
Assessment of technical qualities • Position • Exposure • Inspiratory effort	The X-ray is **straight** if the spinous processes are equidistant from the medial end of each clavicle	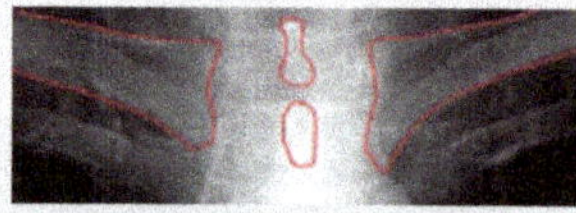
	The **exposure** is adequate if you can see the thoracic spine and intervertebral spaces through the heart	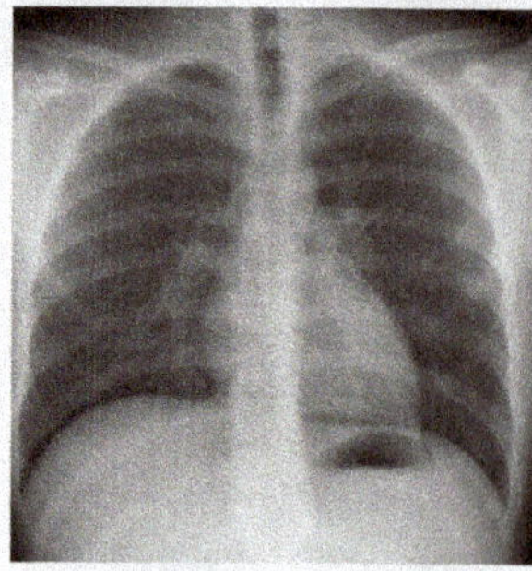
	Inspiratory effort is adequate if 5-6 ribs are visualised on the ventral side and 9-10 ribs on the dorsal side	
Airways • Trachea • Main bronchi	The trachea should be roughly aligned with the midline. The aortic knob usually causes a slight indentation on the left. Tubes should be approx. 2 cm above the carina.	
Bones and soft tissue	Note **positioning**, any **fissures or fractures**, the appearance of the imaged **joints** and any osseous lesions. **Lytic** focal lesions appear as lucent areas, while sclerotic lesions appear as local opaque/dense areas in the bone. **Rib fractures**, with or without dislocation, or **subcutaneous emphysema** (see case image) may be suggestive of other injuries, such as post-traumatic **pneumothorax**.	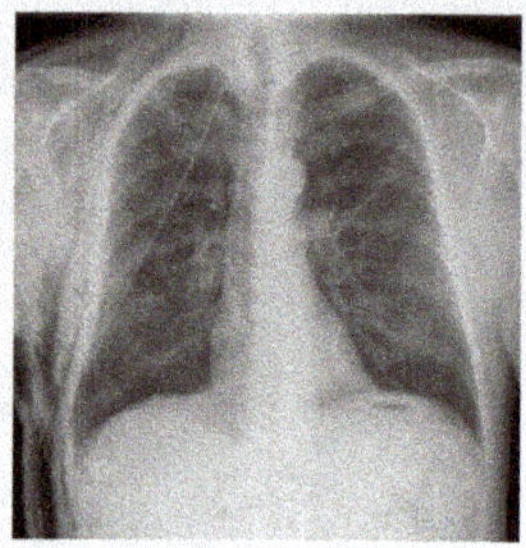

Table 42A // Chest X-ray indications and assessment

EXAM	INDICATIONS	CASE IMAGES
Cardiac and mediastinal silhouette	There is no fixed reference value for mediastinal width, but a width of >85 mm is usually indicative of pathology. A good rule of thumb is that the **left hilum is almost always higher** than the right hilum. Hilar displacement may raise the suspicion that something is pushing or pulling on the hilum. Hilar widening generally results from increased hilar soft tissue (first case image) or dilation of the great vessels (second case image; the arms of the man hiding behind the tree (see dotted line) should not resemble the bodybuilder type). Take a lateral X-ray; enlargement due to hilar masses is easier to see on lateral views.	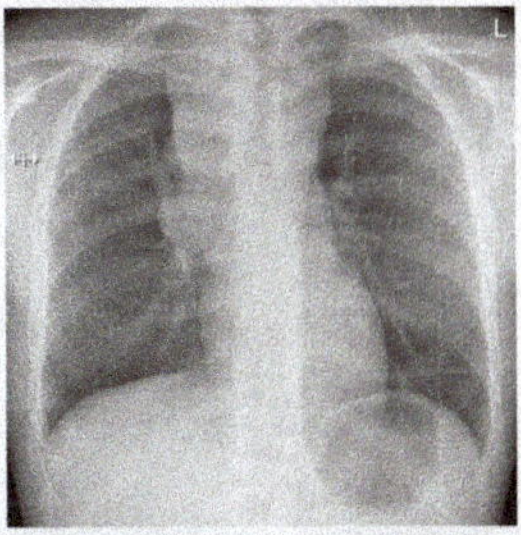 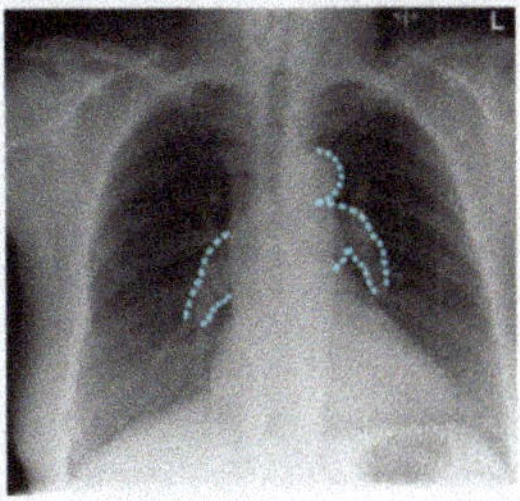

Table 42B // Chest X-ray indications and assessment

In case of suspected intra-abdominal free air, a CT scan is indicated to diagnose perforation of the intestines. On an X-ray, a lucent crescent with sharp edges directly bordering the diaphragm may be seen in the case of intraperitoneal free air (e.g. in the case of massive pneumoperitoneum, the falciform ligament of the liver may be bordered by free air on either side, leading to the appearance of a rugby ball).

EXAM	INDICATIONS	CASE IMAGES
Cardiac and mediastinal silhouette	Generally speaking, cardiomegaly is diagnosed if the maximum diameter of the cardiac silhouette is greater than half the maximum thoracic diameter (third case image, note: AP view). This is also known as cardio-thoracic ratio (CTR), which can only be reliably measured on a posterior-anterior (PA) view. For an AP (antero-posterior) view, an arbitrary cutoff value of 60% can be assumed. When assessing the mediastinum, look closely at the aortopulmonary window too: the space between the aortic knob and the main branch of the left pulmonary artery. There should be air in this window. The presence of (convex) soft tissue in the window may be suggestive of lymphadenopathy or a haematoma, tumour or aneurysm! The **silhouette sign** (referring to a structure that has lost its silhouette) can help detect and localise subtle pathology (see case image, middle lobe consolidation). When interpreting AP/PA views: • Blurred right heart border: middle lobe • Blurred left heart border: lingula • Blurred border of right hemi-diaphragm: right lower lobe • Blurred border of left hemi-diaphragm: left lower lobe • Blurred aortic knob border: upper left lobe	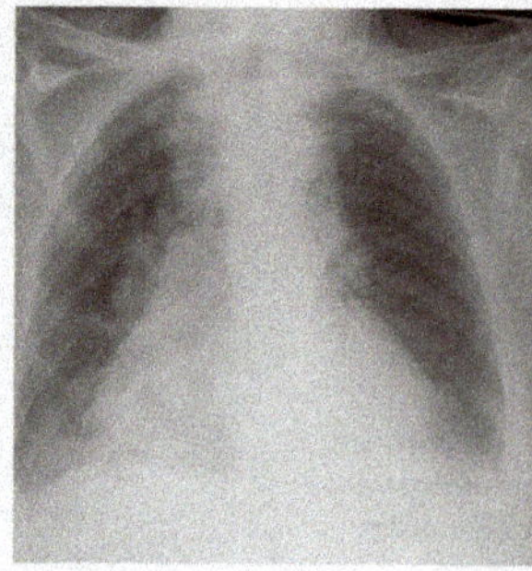 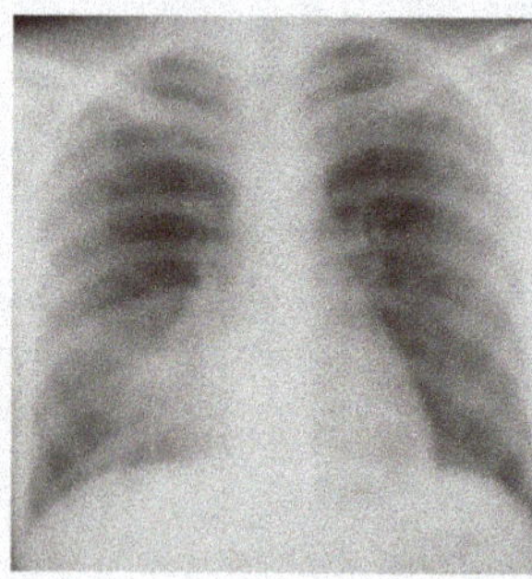

Table 42C // Chest X-ray indications and assessment

EXAM	INDICATIONS	CASE IMAGES
Diaphragm and gastric bubble	The diaphragmal domes are often called **hidden areas**, because pathology in these areas is often overlooked. Generally speaking, the right hemidiaphragm lies higher than the left hemidiaphragm, because it is above the liver (top case image). A **relatively high diaphragm position** may indicate (iatrogenic) phrenic nerve injury, traction due to fibrosis or volume loss of the lung (e.g. after lobectomy). An increase in intra-abdominal pressure may also put pressure on the diaphragm or cause intrathoracic migration of the abdominal viscera (e.g. in a **diaphragmatic hernia**). Note that the projected apex of the diaphragm dome by far does not demarcate the bottom of the lung on PA views (case image). For proper assessment, it is important to also take a lateral X-ray. There is usually gas in the stomach below the left hemidiaphragm (which usually projects as a lucent area over the gastric lumen; see case image). Prominent, air-filled bowel loops may appear under the diaphragm in an ileus. A **standing chest X-ray** may be ordered to assess subdiaphragmatic free air (but preference for a CT scan is increasing). Air rises and spreads out, forming a layer under the diaphragmatic domes.	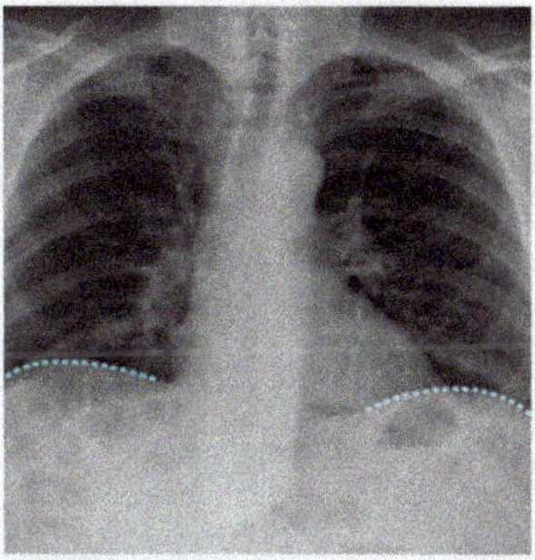 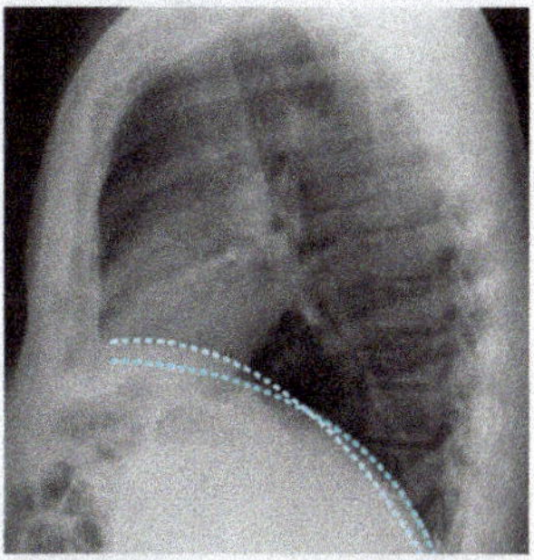 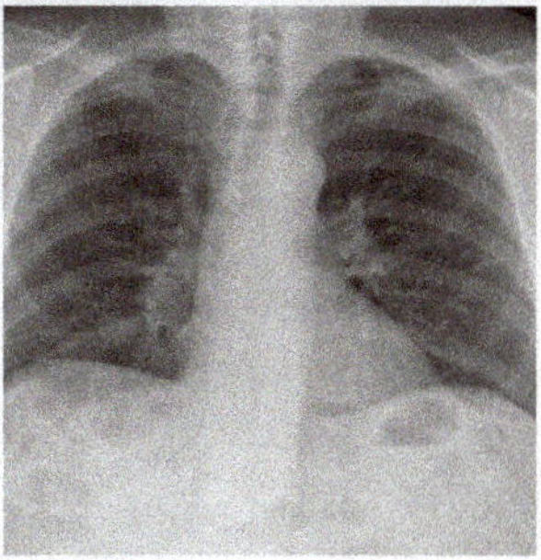

Table 42D // Chest X-ray indications and assessment

On a routine erect chest X-ray, as much as 250-600 ml of pleural fluid may be required for visibility. A lateral or lateral decubitus position may help identify smaller volumes of pleural effusion.

EXAM	INDICATIONS	CASE IMAGES
Effusions	Assessment of the diaphragmatic domes (delineation/position/sub-diaphragmatic abnormalities) also includes assessment of the **pleural sinuses** (usually clearly visible) and **interlobular fissures**. Remember that bilateral pleural fluid may have a very subtle presentation on PA views, manifesting as a slightly rounded sinus. Sometimes abnormalities are obvious, as in the example of left-sided pleural fluid shown here.	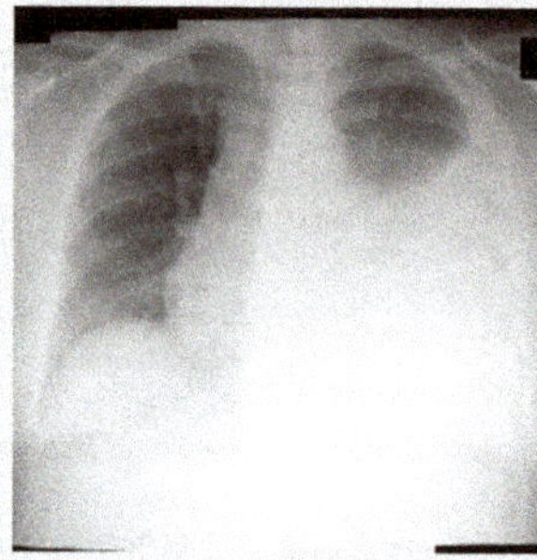
Fields of lungs • RUL: Right Upper Lobe • RLL: Right Lower Lobe • RML: Right Middle Lobe • LUL: Left Upper Lobe • LLL: Left Lower Lobe	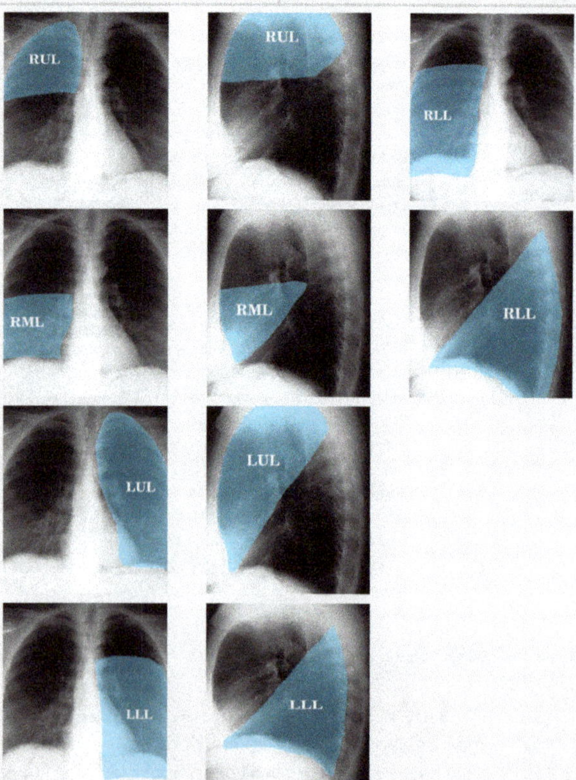	

Table 42E // Chest X-ray indications and assessment

Ultrasonography

In ultrasound, images are acquired using vibrations with frequencies above 20 kHz. Tissue-specific properties (i.e. acoustic impedance) define the degree of absorption (black: anechoic), partial reflection (different shades of grey: hypoechoic to isoechoic), or reflection (white: hyperechoic). For this reason, tissues with similar acoustic impedance (e.g. liver and intrahepatic haemorrhage) may be difficult to distinguish.

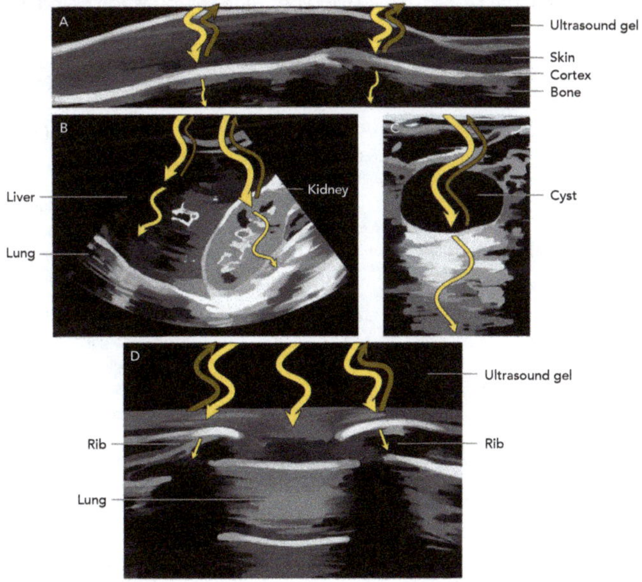

Figure 14 // Different levels of sound wave reflection. The arrows show how much ultrasound is transmitted by the probe into the body. Each tissue type has its own resonance. For example: (A) cortical bone is hyperechoic because of its high/almost full reflectivity, (B) the liver shows different shades of grey due to varying degrees of reflection, (C) fluid in a cyst is not reflective at all, making the contents of the cyst anechoic with posterior wall enhancement, and (D) air looks black due to complete absorption.

Air is disruptive in almost all ultrasound and can result in degraded imaging and suboptimal imaging assessment. Therefore, in an elective setting, patients are advised not to eat prior to an abdominal ultrasound exam.
Exception: absent lung sliding or the barcode sign in M mode are diagnostic indicators of a pneumothorax.

Once air absorbs sound waves entirely, no sound waves will return to the probe; this creates mirror image artefacts. These artefacts are visible on ultrasound as e.g. horizontal lines in the lung or as mirror images of subdiaphragmatic structures (such as the liver and spleen).

Point of care ultrasonography (POCUS)

Interpretation of POCUS depends on the combination of imaging in multiple planes, clinical findings, and the question being asked.

EXAM	INDICATIONS	ASSESSMENT
Extended (e)FAST	• High-energy trauma (HET) • Sharp/blunt force trauma to the abdomen, flanks, and/or thorax • Haemodynamically unstable patient with unclear aetiology	1. Pneumothorax (absence of pleural sliding) 2. Pleural fluid 3. Pericardial fluid 4. Intra-abdominal free fluid (around the liver, spleen, hepatorenal recess, rectovesical pouch/rectouterine pouch) 5. Abdominal aorta (aneurysm, intimal flap)
Lung	• Shortness of breath • Pneumonia • Pleural effusion • Empyema • (Cardiogenic) pulmonary oedema • Acute respiratory distress syndrome (ARDS) • Pneumothorax	1. Pneumothorax (pleural sliding, lung pulse sign, lung point sign) 2. Aerated lung (A-lines, pleural sliding) 3. Interstitial fluid (B-lines) 4. (Subpleural) consolidations 5. Pleural effusion 6. Diaphragm function
Heart	• Cardiac arrest • Acute decompensated HF • Clinical suspicion of cardiac tamponade • Pulmonary embolism	1. Global left ventricular function 2. Right ventricular overload (D sign, protusion of septum in the left ventricle (LV)) 3. Pericardial effusion 4. Estimated RA pressure to evaluate volume status (see VCI)
Kidneys and bladder	• Flank pain • Acute renal insufficiency • Pyelonephritis • Anuria	1. Shape and size of kidneys 2. Homogeneity parenchyma 3. Hydronephrosis 4. Kidney stones 5. Perirenal free fluid 6. Aspect bladder and contents 7. Position possible catheters (e.g. nephrostomy, JJ-catheter, bladder catheter)

Table 43A // POCUS

EXAM	INDICATIONS	ASSESSMENT
Vena cava inferior (VCI)	• Volume status • Shock • Shortness of breath	1. Diameter VCI 2 cm from inlet right atrium (RA) 2. Diameter and degree of collapse of the VCI 3. Estimated RA pressure
Duplex/ doppler	• DVT • Thrombophlebitis	1. Thrombus (isoechoic intravascular structus) 2. Non-compressible 3. Absence of flow

Table 43B // POCUS

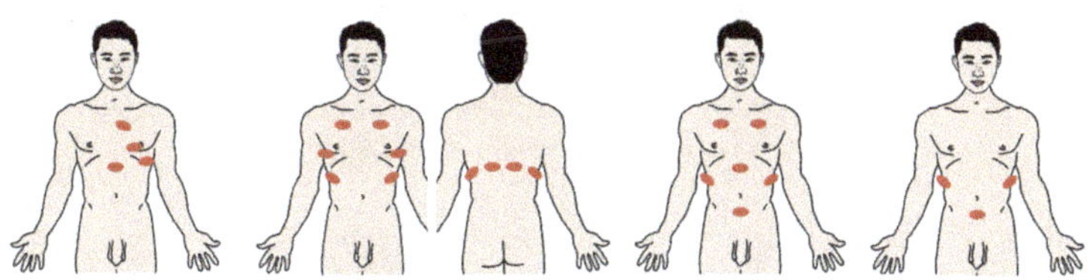

Figure 15 // POCUS of the heart (A), lungs (B), eFAST (C), and kidneys and bladder (D).

In POCUS B-lines represent pathology and are non-specific. They can be seen in interstitial fluid, emphysema, pneumonia and COPD-like disorders.

Computed tomography (CT)

Comparable to the X-ray technique, CT uses X-rays (photons) to create 3D images. Images are initially made in the axial plane. When the exam is finished, reconstructions can also be made in other planes (e.g. coronal, sagittal).

When performing a CT patients can be scanned several times while using iodinated contrast agents, creating multiple scan phases (see Tables 44-47). Contrast agents are hyperdense (whiter) on CT scans, making them easily identifiable. Iodinated contrast is virtually the only type of IV contrast used for CT scans. Iodine has a high atomic number, which means it blocks more X-rays than the other structures on the image – for example, it is easier to distinguish the lumen of blood vessels on a scan; organs absorbing iodinated contrast at that moment (e.g. liver, spleen, kidneys) become denser on a scan; and insufficiently perfused tissue will be less dense. How tissues and blood vessels are visualised depends on the phase in which they are scanned. In CT angiography (CTA) or CT venography (CTV), the patient is scanned when the contrast agent is in the artery or the vein, respectively. This is combined with knowledge of tissue physiology to detect pathology.

Non-contrast CT and contrast CT are two examples of scan protocols. In contrast CTs there are many different scan phases to choose from. For this reason radiologists need a clear, detailed imaging request to determine the optimal scan phase to provide an answer to the clinical dilemma.

Scan phases refer to the location of iodinated contrast agents used in CT imaging to better assess organs and anatomic structures. Depending on the target organ or clinical dilemma multiple scan phases may be required.

Bones

TEST		INDICATIONS	ASSESSMENT
Skeletal CT	**Without contrast**	• Fractures of the extremities/spine: preoperative planning, assessment of complexity • Tumours/metastases (when MRI is contraindicated) • Spinal stenosis/radiculopathy (when MRI is contraindicated)	• Main imaged osseous structure: cortical delineation, joint juxtaposition (degree of dislocation, lysis/listhesis in vertebral bodies, vertebral discs/cartilage), bone density (osteoporosis/lytic or sclerotic lesions) • Other osseous structures on image • Soft-tissue swelling

Table 44 // Indications for and assessment of skeletal CT

Head-neck

TEST		INDICATIONS	ASSESSMENT
Head-neck CT	**Without contrast**	• Haemorrhage (epidural, subdural, subarachnoid, parenchymal) • Infarction • Suspected herniation/ mass effect	• Ventricles: symmetry, dilatation, compression, intraventricular blood • Brain parenchyma: gyri/sulci (asymmetry or obliteration), midline shift, grey-white matter differentiation, atrophy/ischaemia of different brain lobes, brainstem, cerebellum, basal ganglia, thalamus, hypothalamus, pituitary gland • Subarachnoid cisterns: evidence of SAH • Bones: skull, facial structures, aeration of sinus and mastoid

Table 45A // Indications for and assessment of head-neck CT

TEST		INDICATIONS	ASSESSMENT
Head-neck CT	With contrast	• Thrombosis (arterial, venous/sinus) and ischaemia (perfusion: penumbra and core infarction) • Aneurysms • Arteriovenous malformations (AVM) • Intracranial tumour • Infection/abscess • Risk of airway compromise (e.g. neck tumours)	• Arteries: common carotid artery, external carotid artery, internal carotid artery, vertebral artery, basilar artery, anterior cerebral artery, anterior communicating artery, middle cerebral artery, posterior cerebral artery, posterior communicating artery, circle of Willis • Veins: superior sagittal sinus, straight sinus, transverse sinus, sigmoid sinus, cavernous sinus, internal jugular vein, external jugular vein • Contrast enhancement of intracranial structures/pathology

Table 45B // Indications for and assessment of head-neck CT

Chest

TEST		INDICATIONS	ASSESSMENT
Chest CT	Without contrast	• Pathology affecting the lung parenchyma • Trauma (lung, fractures)	• Organs: trachea, oesophagus, lungs, heart (atria, ventricles, septum, pericardium), diaphragm • Bones: sternum, ribs, scapulae, glenohumeral joint, acromioclavicular (AC) and sternoclavicular joint, spine
	With contrast	Supplement or alternative to non-contrast chest CT: • Suspected pulmonary embolism, aortic dissection, aortic anomalies • Cancer staging (e.g. lung malignancies) • Mediastinal pathology (e.g. lymphadenopathy, thymus pathology) • Postoperative complications (e.g. mediastinal haematoma, fluid collections)	• Lymph nodes • Upper abdominal organs • Arteries and veins: aorta, vessels originating from the aortic arc (subclavian artery, carotid artery, brachiocephalic trunk), superior/inferior vena cava, subclavian vein, pulmonary trunk, pulmonary vein/artery, coronary arteries

Table 46 // Indications for and assessment of chest CT

Abdomen

TEST		INDICATIONS	ASSESSMENT
Abdominal CT	Without contrast	Kidney/ureteric stones	• Kidneys (cortex and renal pelvis), ureter, bladder • Other: basal lung fields, diaphragm, heart (atria, ventricles, septum, pericardium), adrenal glands • Bones: ribs, vertebrae, pelvis, femoral head
	With contrast		

Table 47A // Indications for and assessment of abdominal CT

	TEST	INDICATIONS	ASSESSMENT
Abdominal CT	**CT angiography (CTA)**	• Abdominal bleeding • Aortic aneurysm • Arterial stenoses/occlusions • Hypervascular (liver) metastases • Pancreatic tumours	• Organs: liver (intrahepatic bile ducts), gallbladder and extrahepatic bile ducts, pancreas, spleen, kidneys • Digestive tract: oesophagus, stomach, antrum, duodenum, jejunum, ileum, colon (e.g. caecum, appendix), sigmoid, rectum • Portal system: mesenteric vein (superior and inferior), splenic vein, hepatic vein, portal vein • Arteries: aorta, coeliac trunk, mesenteric artery (superior and inferior), renal artery, common/internal/external iliac artery, common, superficial/deep femoral artery • Veins: inferior vena cava, renal vein, femoral vein, iliac vein, mesenteric vein, splenic vein, hepatic vein, portal vein • Other: lymphadenopathy, ascites, musculature • Fat infiltration
	CT portal venography (CTV)	• General screening for abdominal pathology • Hypovascular (liver) metastases • Abscess formation • Venous thrombosis	
	Nephrogenic	• Kidney tumours • Kidney trauma	
	Equilibrium delayed (wash-out phase)	• Ureteral obstruction or leakage • Tumours of the abdominal organs	

Table 47B // Indications for and assessment of abdominal CT

CT perfusion (CTP)

A CTP is a CT scan of the brain that uses iodine contrast to calculate the perfusion of brain tissue based on different flow parameters. After IV administration of iodine contrast cerebral blood flow (CBF), cerebral blood volume (CBV) and mean transit time (MTT) are calculated and displayed in different colours. Depending on the software, red areas represent high perfusion and blue areas represent low perfusion. Based on these series the infarct core (unsalvageable tissue) and penumbra (salvageable tissue) of an ischaemic stroke are calculated. Mostly, the core is displayed in red and the penumbra in green (see Figure 16). A CTP is used in most centres in addition to a non-contrast brain CT and CTA to increase the diagnostic accuracy for the indication of acute interventions in ischaemic strokes.

> Inaccurate perfusion maps may be due to cardiovascular disease (e.g. a poor cardiac output, atrial fibrillation (AF), severe arterial stenosis) or inadequate placement of regions of interest (e.g. arterial and venous density regions).

- If the penumbra is larger than the core (mismatch), IVT can be administered up to 12h after stroke onset and mechanical thrombectomy can be executed up to 24h after onset.
- Note that the exact time window for 'late' IVT and thrombectomy differs worldwide, therefore always consult the local guidelines in acute treatment of an ischaemic stroke.

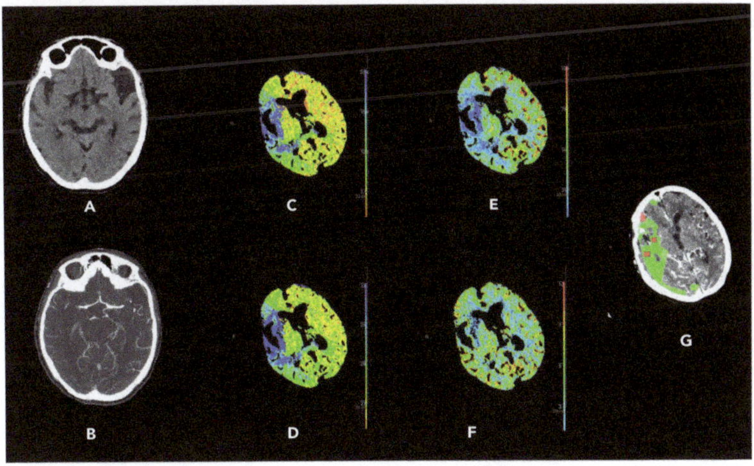

Figure 16 // CT perfusion with a defect in the right MCA supply area

A: Brain CT without contrast. **B:** CTA showing an occlusion of the right middle cerebral artery with **C:** increased MTT, **D:** increased time to peak (TTP), **E:** decreased CBF, and **F:** decreased CBV of the affected area. **G:** Calculated perfusion with large penumbra in right hemisphere (green) and no evident infarct core (red).

MRI is generally not used in an emergency setting, however, it should be considered in the following situations:

- Suspicion of an intraspinal (epidural) haemorrhage or unstable spinal fracture where surgical intervention may be indicated
- Suspicion of intracranial complications of an infection (e.g. meningitis, encephalitis), esp. in children (in emergency settings often following a primary head CT)
- Suspected hydrocephalus in children
- Clinical cauda syndrome

There are certain indications that require a semi-acute MRI, such as a hypoxic-ischemic event in children.

Pharmacological treatment

Legend

- ☼ = Additional information
- ● = Indication for prescribing medication
- ⇔ = Interaction with drugs or high-risk groups
- ⊗ = Indication for stopping with medication
- ▲ = Intoxication management

Pain management

Pain is an unpleasant sensation and emotional experience that is often, but not always, associated with actual or potential tissue damage. There are three different types of pain including nociceptive pain, neuropathic pain and nociplastic pain.

Nociceptive pain

D Nociceptive pain arises from actual damage or risk of damage to non-neural tissue.

Ae Trauma, inflammation, infection, surgery

Hx Sharp and localised pain (e.g. wound, somatic, parietal), dull, gnawing and less localised (visceral), or perceived at a location other than the site of the painful stimulus (referred pain)

Tx Treatment of the underlying cause

Physical therapy, relaxation techniques

- Analgesics following the WHO analgesic ladder (see Table 48)
- Locoregional interventions such as epidural and peripheral nerve blocks

Neuropathic pain

D Neuropathic pain is caused by a lesion or disease of the peripheral and/or central nervous system (CNS).

R Advanced age, ♀, pre-operative and post-operative pain, obesity, anxiety, catastrophising

Ae Spinal cord injury, limb amputation, stroke, multiple sclerosis, herniated disc, DM, metabolic disorder, herpes zoster, chemotherapy, radiation, cancer, nerve lesion, burn wound, trauma, surgery, polyneuropathy

Hx Triggered and/or spontaneous pain. Burning, painful cold, electric shock, tingling, pins and needles, numbness, itching (DN4 criteria), muscle weakness.

PE Hypoesthesia, anaesthesia, hypoalgesia, hyperalgesia, dysesthesia, allodynia in area supplied by nerve, decreased motor function

Dx
- Classic nerve conduction study: prolonged distal latency ↑, conduction velocity ↓, and F-wave latency ↑ in demyelinating injury
- Electromyography (EMG): positive sharp waves and fibrillations at rest and during voluntary activity indicate denervation from axonal loss (not present in demyelinating-type polyneuropathy)
- Spinal MRI: identify cause and level of potential nerve root entrapment or myelum compression

Tx Mirror therapy for phantom pain, physical therapy for herniated disc, music therapy for burn wound care

Antidepressant (e.g. amitriptyline, nortriptyline), anticonvulsant (e.g. pregabalin, gabapentin, carbamazepine), SNRI (e.g. duloxetine, venlafaxine) and/or transdermal patch of lidocaine/capsaicin in consultation with a pain specialist. Effect after 2-3 wk, side effects are often the worst during first 2 wk.

Nociplastic pain

D Nociplastic pain arises from altered nociception, despite clear evidence of the absence of actual or threatened tissue damage or evidence for disease/lesion of the nervous system, assumed to be caused by central sensitisation.

R Stress, disability, depression, sleep disturbance, obesity, sexual abuse, anxiety, catastrophising

Ae Associated with different chronic pain syndromes such as chronic widespread pain, fibromyalgia, chronic pelvic pain syndrome, chronic low back pain, migraine, irritable bowel syndrome (IBS)

Hx Widespread pain, fluctuates in location and intensity. Psychological symptoms such as fatigue, depression, anxiety and catastrophizing. Social symptoms such as isolation, loneliness, financial difficulties and loss of job. Spiritual symptoms such as loss of faith and meaning of life.

PE Widespread, not following a specific nerve or dermatome, hypoalgesia, hyperalgesia, allodynia

Dx Quantitative sensory testing

Tx Multidisciplinary approach (e.g. pain education, healthy lifestyle, psychological therapies, anti-neuropathic drugs, pain rehabilitation) in consultation with pain specialist

Avoid opioids

- **Hypoalgesia:** diminished pain in response to a normally painful stimulus.
- **Hyperalgesia:** increased responsiveness of nociceptive neurons in the CNS to their normal or subthreshold afferent input (e.g. pin-prick).
- **Allodynia:** pain due to a stimulus that does not normally provoke pain (e.g. brushing).
- **Dysesthesia:** an unpleasant abnormal sensation, whether spontaneous or evoked.
- **Hypoesthesia:** diminished ability to perceive pain, temperature, touch, or vibration.
- **Anaesthesia:** complete inability to perceive pain, temperature, touch, or vibration.
- **Central sensitisation:** increased responsiveness of nociceptive neurons in the CNS to their normal or subthreshold afferent input.

Naloxone is an opioid antagonist.
Mechanism of action: Competitive opioid receptor (μ, δ and κ-receptor) antagonist
Indications:
- Reversing respiratory/CNS depression caused by opioid use
- Treatment in (suspected) overdose/intoxication of opioids

Adverse effects:
- Nausea and/or vomiting
- Headache, dizziness, tachycardia

Notes: Risk of cardiac arrest, VT and VF in patients with tricyclic antidepressants, calcium antagonists, beta blockers or digoxin

Opioids:

- To prevent constipation, always prescribe opioids together with an osmotic laxative such as macrogol or magnesium.
- Start with SC or IV administration (e.g. patient controlled anaesthesia (PCA) pump) if a quick effect is desired or if the patient is not able to swallow by mouth or has poor gut absorption.
- Prescribe opioids for a short period and at the lowest dosage possible because of tolerance, addiction, and nausea.
- Always choose a long-acting opioid together with a short-acting (1/6 of the equivalent long-acting dose per day) for breakthrough pain. Increase the dose of the long-acting opioid when the short-acting opioid is used more than three times a day.

Cancer pain:

- Often a combination of nociceptive and neuropathic pain due to tumour ingrowth, chemotherapy, radiation, and surgery.
- Consider radiotherapy, bisphosphate, and/or NSAID in case of bone pain caused by osteolytic metastases.
- Consider invasive interventions such as neurolytic blocks and epidurals or intrathecal catheters in consultation with a pain specialist.

Analgesics

Use an opioid calculator for adequate dosage when rotating/changing opioids.

When rotating to methadone or buprenorphine, a pain specialist should always be consulted.

When converting from one opioid to another, the calculated 24h dose should be reduced by 25-50% depending on the level of pain the individual experiences at that time.

STEP		MEDICATION	MECHANISM OF ACTION
1	**Start paracetamol**	Paracetamol	Unclear
2	**Add NSAID**	Diclofenac	COX-1 and 2 inhibition
		Ibuprofen	
		Naproxen	
		Ketorolac	
		Etoricoxib/celecoxib	COX-2 inhibition
		Metamizole	COX-1 and 2 inhibition, possible COX-3 inhibition
3 (optional)	**Add weak opioid**	Codeine	Prodrug with unpredictable conversion to morphine (10x less potent)
		Tramadol	Weak agonist of MOP and SNRI/SSRI
4	**Replace weak opioid with strong opioid**	Morphine	Full agonist of three opioid receptors (MOP, KOP, DOP) and SNRI/SSRI
		Oxycodone	
		Fentanyl	
		Buprenorphine	Partial agonist of MOP and antagonist of KOP

Table 48A // WHO analgesic ladder

ADVERSE EFFECTS	NOTES
Mild adverse effect profile: risk of liver damage at high doses (>150 mg/kg) and in cases of alcoholism and pre-existing liver damage	💡 Administer lower dosage in malnutrition, active alcohol abuse, weight <50 kg ⊗ CI: liver failure
• GI: risk of peptic ulcer • Renal: peripheral oedema, acute/chronic renal insufficiency especially in patients on RAS inhibitors, diuretics, pre-existing renal insufficiency, HF, dehydration, sepsis • Cardiovascular: potential potassium risk esp. with COX-2 inhibitors and diclofenac, including risk of HF	💡 Diclofenac has the highest CV risk and naproxen/ketorolac the highest GI risk. NSAIDs can cause acute renal failure when combined with ACE inhibitors and diuretics and all increase the risk of bleeding. ⇔ Prescribe prophylactic dose of PPI to patients aged >70, peptic ulcer in PMHx, or age >60 with DM, rheumatoid arthritis, HF or use of corticosteroids, SSRIs, OAC, or acetylsalicylic acid ⊗ CI: peptic ulcer, inflammatory bowel disease, renal and liver failure, HF, cardiovascular disease, pregnancy
	💡 Fewer renal and GI adverse effects, but higher CV risk than classic NSAIDs
	💡 Less kidney, CV, and GI toxicity than classic NSAIDs ⊗ Agranulocytosis is a very rare side effect, monitor CBC when prescribing for longer period ⊗ CI: agranulocytosis, bone marrow disorder, G6PD deficiency, porphyria, renal failure
• CNS: respiratory depression (esp. high-risk in COPD), miosis, delirium, sedation, dependence • Pulmonary: bronchoconstriction • GI: motility ↓ (constipation, nausea, vomiting)	💡 Up to 10% of the North European and American population may be poor metabolisers and up to 10% may be ultra-rapid metabolisers
	⇔ When combined with drugs affecting serotonin (e.g. SSRI, MAO inhibitors) → risk of serotonin syndrome ↑ CI: Severe COPD and asthma (bronchoconstriction), severe OSAS, intracranial injury, renal and liver failure, neuromuscular disease
	⇔ Risk of respiratory depression and sedation with alcoholism, renal failure, advanced age and CNS depressants (anxiolytics, antidepressants, sedatives)
	💡 Preferred opioid for patients with renal failure. Fentanyl is available for transdermal (effect after ±12h), buccal, sublingual, and intranasal administration (effect after several min).
	💡 Less likely to cause addiction because of its partial agonist activity. Do not prescribe together with other opioids. Buprenorphine is available for transdermal (effect after ±12h) and sublingual administration.

STEP		MEDICATION	MECHANISM OF ACTION
5	**Consult the APS in your hospital for other options** (e.g. opioid rotation, (es)ketamine/ lidocaine infusion, methadone)	Calculate the oral morphine equivalents per 24h, and reduce the dose of the new opioid to 75% of the previous opioid.	

Table 48B // WHO analgesic ladder

APS, acute pain service; CNS, central nervous system; CBC, complete blood count; COX, cyclo-oxygenase; CV, cardiovascular; GI, gastrointestinal; DOP, delta opioid peptide receptor; M6G, morphine-6-glucuronide; MOP, mu opioid peptide receptor; KOP, kappa opioid peptide receptor; OSAS, obstructive sleep apnoea syndrome; SSRI, selective serotonin reuptake inhibitors; SNRI, selective noradrenaline reuptake inhibitors; PPI, proton pump inhibitor

Anticoagulants

	MEDICATION	MECHANISM OF ACTION	INDICATIONS
PLATELET AGGREGATION INHIBITORS	**Acetylsalicylic acid**	ASA irreversibly inhibits the COX enzyme (→ production of platelet aggregation-stimulating thromboxane A2 ↓)	Treatment of ACS, AP and PAD, treatment of MI, CABG, TIA, and ischaemic stroke
	P2Y12 inhibitors (e.g. clopidogrel, prasugrel, ticagrelor)	P2Y12 inhibitors irreversibly inhibit activation via the ADP receptor on the platelet	ACS, TIA or ischaemic stroke. Often used in combination with ASA as dual antiplatelet therapy (DAPT).
	Glycoprotein IIb/IIIa inhibitors (e.g. abciximab, tirofiban, eptifibatide)	Glycoprotein IIb/IIIa receptor inhibition → inhibits binding fibrinogen and von Willebrand Factor → platelet aggregation ↓	Acute coronary syndromes
VKA	**Vitamin K antagonists** (e.g. acenocoumarol, phenprocoumon, warfarin)	Inhibition of vitamin K and with it the synthesis of coagulation factors II/VII/IX/X: • Acenocoumarol has a $t_{1/2}$ of 8-11h, an onset of action of 36-72h and a duration of action of 2d • Phenprocoumon has a $t_{1/2}$ of 160h, an onset of action of 48-72h and a duration of action of 1-2wk	Indicated for: • AF (CHA_2DS_2-VA >1) • Mechanical valve prosthesis • Venous thromboembolism (DVT, pulmonary embolism); duration: 3 mo (1st VTE episode provoked by transient risk factor), 6 mo (first idiopathic VTE), >1y (recurring VTE)

Table 49A // Anticoagulants

ADVERSE EFFECTS	NOTES
Calculate the oral morphine equivalents per 24h, and reduce the dose of the new opioid to 75% of the previous opioid.	

ADVERSE EFFECTS	NOTES
• Hypersensitivity (urticaria, exanthema, angioedema) • Bleeding risk ↑ (haematoma, epistaxis, GI bleeding) • GI (stomach problems)	⇔ Bleeding risk in the elderly and patients using corticosteroids, other NSAIDs and SSRIs ↑ ⊗ Prior to procedures with a high risk of bleeding complications, such as neurosurgery: stop ASA/clopidogrel 5-7d in advance. Due to irreversible binding, the duration of action of both drugs is 3-10d. ● Perioperative platelet transfusion in case of acute haemorrhage secondary to ASA or clopidogrel use
• Bleeding risk ↑ (haematoma, epistaxis, GI bleeding) • abdominal pain, diarrhoea, dyspepsia	
• Bleeding risk ↑ • Thrombocytopenia	● Can be indicated after PCI in the case of no/inadequate reperfusion
Bleeding risk ↑	⇔ Bleeding risk ↑ due to: • Corticosteroids and NSAIDs (ulcerogenic) • SSRIs combined with platelet aggregation inhibitor (thrombocytopathy) • Nonadherence • Alcohol consumption • Low vitamin K intake • Febrile illness • Enhanced action of VKA due to cotrimoxazole or after sudden discontinuation of carbamazepine or rifampicin 💡 For haemorrhage management: see following pages

	MEDICATION	MECHANISM OF ACTION	INDICATIONS
HEPARIN GROUP	**Factor Xa inhibitors** (e.g. fondaparinux)	Binding to antithrombin III → factor Xa inhibition	Used to treat venous and arterial thromboembolic disorders before starting OAC, also used as prophylaxis for surgical patients and for bridging. Therapeutic (6 mo) in VTE secondary to malignancy.
	Heparin	Heparin (SC/IV) activates antithrombin (factor III) and thus indirectly inactivates factors Xa and IIa (thrombin)	
	LMWH (e.g. nadroparin, enoxaparin)	LMWHs SC contain fragments of heparin with higher anti-Xa activity and lower anti-IIa activity. LMWHs are renally cleared.	
DOAC	**Direct IIa inhibitors** (e.g. dagibatran)	Competitive and reversible inhibition of activated factor II	• Prevention of stroke and systemic embolism in nonvalvular atrial fibrillation • Treatment of DVT and pulmonary embolism and prevention of recurrent VTE • DOACs can not be used as anticoagulant for mechanical heart valves, and moderate to severe mitral valve stenosis
	Factor Xa inhibitors (e.g. rivaroxaban, apixaban, edoxaban)	Selective inhibition of activated factor X	

Table 49B // Anticoagulants

ACS, acute coronary syndrome; ADP, adenosine diphosphate; AF, atrial fibrillation; AP, angina pectoris; CABG, coronary artery bypass graft; DOAC, direct oral anticoagulants; DVT, deep vein thrombosis; LMWH, low-molecular-weight heparin; OAC, oral anticoagulation; PAD, peripheral arterial disease; PCI, percutaneous coronary intervention; Pgp, P-glycoprotein; TIA, transient ischaemic attack; VKA, vitamin K antagonists; VTE, venous thromboembolism

All antiplatelet drugs require an initial loading dose, often higher, followed by a lower maintenance dose for continued treatment.

The efficacy of **vitamin K antagonists** (coumarin derivatives) depends on the INR. In case of haemorrhage or INR overshoots, vitamin K can be given orally (effect >8h) or intravenously (>6h). Vitamin K treatment lasts 24h and must be repeated, certainly with phenprocoumon (long $t_{1/2}$). In life-threatening situations like intracranial haemorrhages a four-factor prothrombin complex concentrate (II, VII, IX, X) should also be administered.

ADVERSE EFFECTS	NOTES
• Bleeding risk ↑ • Heparin-induced thrombocytopenia (HIT) type I/II • Anaphylaxis • Transaminases ↑	Bridging: before any invasive procedure with bleeding risk, a short-acting medication (LMWH/ heparin) is administered to bridge the discontinuation of the OAC Following acute haemorrhaging, discontinue heparin/LMWH and administer protamine (partially inhibits anti-Xa activity, less so with LMWH!) IV as an antidote For more information on therapeutic blood monitoring, see the following pages
• Bleeding risk ↑ • Anaemia • GI: dyspepsia, diarrhoea, nausea, vomiting • Kidney function ↓	⇔ Bleeding risk ↑: • Corticosteroids and NSAIDs • Platelet aggregation inhibitors combined with SSRIs • Thrombolytics • Nonadherence • Alcohol consumption • Febrile illness • Pgp inhibitors such as ciclosporin, itraconazole, ketoconazole, amiodarone and verapamil In case of active haemorrhaging on dabigatran, idaruzicimab can be administered as an antidote. In case of direct Xa inhibitors, andexanet alpha can be administered.

LMWHs have a longer $t_{1/2}$ and more stable serum levels, and no anti-Xa activity monitoring is needed. In case of reduced LMWH renal clearance, the dose should be adjusted based on anti-Xa levels.

DOACs are taken orally and do not require routine INR monitoring, reducing patient burden. DOAC treatment is as effective as VKA treatment, with comparable risk of stroke, cardiovascular death, and other causes of mortality. DOACs are additionally associated with a reduced risk of major bleeding, including intracranial bleeding, compared to VKAs.

DOACs are not indicated in patients with mechanical heart valves. These patients should be treated with vitamin K antagonists.

INR

The international normalised ratio (INR) is the rate at which blood clots. The physiological INR is 1. An INR of 2 means that blood clots twice as slowly. The target value of INR is between 2.0-3.5, depending on the thrombotic risk.

Bridging

Bridging involves temporarily administering a short-acting agent (LMWH or occasionally unfractionated heparin) to bridge the time without VKA. Coumarin derivatives must be discontinued prior to any invasive procedure with a high bleeding risk. Due to their respective elimination half-lives, acenocoumarol should be discontinued three to four days and phenprocoumon five to seven days prior to surgery.

Bridging is indicated in patients with an increased risk of thrombosis. This risk can be estimated with the CHA_2DS_2-VA score, which uses validated risk factors to evaluate ischaemic stroke risk in patients with AF. Preoperative discontinuation of DOACs is not an indication for bridging because of the short $t_{1/2}$.

Bridging with LMWH is indicated for:

- Very high arterial thromboembolism risk: AF with CHA_2DS_2-VA score 8-9, mechanical or bioprosthetic heart valve, or a stroke/TIA <6 months ago.
- Very high venous thromboembolism (VTE) risk: <3 months after first or recurrent idiopathic DVT/pulmonary embolism.

Diuretics

	MEDICATION	MECHANISM OF ACTION	INDICATIONS
DIURETICS	**Acetazolamide**	Carboanhydrase inhibitor → renal HCO_3^- and Na^+ excretion ↑	• HF • High altitude sickness • Increased intracranial pressure • Glaucoma
	Loop diuretics (e.g. furosemide, bumetanide, torasemide)	Loop diuretics inhibit Na^+-K^+-$2Cl^-$ cotransporters in the loop of Henle. Thiazide diuretics inhibit Na^+-Cl^- cotransporters further downstream in the distal tubule, leading to increased Na^+ absorption at the expense of K^+ absorption.	• Oedematous disease (HF, liver cirrhosis, nephrotic syndrome) • Acute hypercalcaemia • Hypertension with a GFR <30 ml/min
	Thiazide diuretics (e.g. hydrochlorothiazide (HCT), chlorthalidone)		• Hypertension • Mild oedema (HF NYHA II/III, nephrotic syndrome, liver cirrhosis) • Nephrogenic diabetes insipidus

Table 50A // Diuretics

The CHA_2DS_2-VA score:

Congestive HF	1 point
Hypertension	1 point
Age ≥75	2 points
Diabetes mellitus	1 point
Stroke/TIA/arterial thromboembolism	2 points
Vascular disease	1 point
Age 65-74	1 point

The **HAS-BLED** Score can be used to assess bleeding risk.

Criterium	**Points**
Hypertension	1 point
Abnormal renal or liver function	1 point each
Stroke	1 point
Bleeding	1 point
Labile INRs	1 point
Elderly (>65)	1 point
Drugs or alcohol	1 point each

ADVERSE EFFECTS	NOTES
• Bone marrow depression • Anaphylaxis • Rash • Electrolyte disorders	⇔ Oral anticoagulants, diabetes mellitus medication
• Volume depletion (orthostatic hypotension, dehydration especially in the elderly), hyperuricaemia/gout • Hypokalaemia (arrhythmias, muscle weakness) • Interference with other electrolytes (Na^+, Mg^{2+}, H^+)	Increase the dose of the loop diuretic in patients with renal insufficiency (more effective than thiazide diuretics at GFR <30 ml/min)
• Orthostatic hypotension (risk of falling, dizziness) • Hypokalaemia (arrhythmias, muscle weakness) • Hyponatraemia (nausea, confusion, risk of falling)	⇔ Hyponatraemia secondary to thiazide diuretics is particularly common in elderly patients. Monitor Na^+ levels 5-9d after starting treatment/increasing the dose (patients aged ≥70 + SSRI, NSAIDs, carbamazepine or loop diuretic or if aged ≥80).

	MEDICATION	MECHANISM OF ACTION	INDICATIONS
DIURETICS	**Mineralocorticoid receptor antagonists (MRA)** (e.g. spironolactone, eplerenone, amiloride, triamterene)	Spironolactone and eplerenone inhibit Na^+-K^+ exchange by blocking aldosterone receptors. Amiloride and triamterene block the epithelial Na^+ channel in the collecting duct	• Adjuvant against hypokalaemia when taking loop and thiazide diuretics • Oedema due to HF NYHA III or liver cirrhosis • Hyperaldosteronism (spironolactone)
	Selective sodium-glucose transporter-2 (SGLT2) inhibitors (e.g. dapagliflozin, empagliflozin)	• Glucose reabsorption ↓ → renal glucose excretion ↑ • Sodium reabsorption ↓ → natriuresis ↑ → preload ↓ • Vasodilation → afterload ↓	• HFrEF, HFpEF • Cardiac patients with diabetes mellitus

Table 50B // Diuretics

ACE, angiotensin-converting enzyme; ARBs, angiotensin receptor blockers; NYHA, New York Heart Association Classification

For hypokalaemia, an MRA or a low-dose ACE inhibitor can be added. Check K^+ level before starting treatment and again <1-2 wk in patients aged >80 or high-risk patients aged >70.

Beta blockers

	MEDICATION	MECHANISM OF ACTION	INDICATIONS
BETA BLOCKERS	**Selective β1 receptor blockers** (e.g. metoprolol, bisoprolol, nebivolol)	Beta receptor blockade: BP ↓, CO ↓ (HR ↓ and SV ↑), cardiac contractility ↑ and bronchoconstriction. β1 receptors reside in myocardial pacemaker cells; β2 receptors are peripheral, located in airways and blood vessels	• Ischemic heart disease • Hypertension • AF (rate and rhythm (sotalol) control) • Secondary prevention after acute MI • Stable chronic HF (EF <35%)
	Non-selective β1 and β2 receptor blockers (e.g. sotalol, propanolol)		

Table 51 // Beta blockers

BP, blood pressure; CO, cardiac output; EF, ejection fraction; HR, heart rate; SV, stroke volume

Labetalol and carvedilol also have an alfa-receptor mediated effect.

ADVERSE EFFECTS	NOTES
• Hyperkalaemia • Nausea • Gynaecomastia and libido ↓ (spironolactone)	⇔ Risk of hyperkalaemia ↑ in DM, renal failure, HF, ACE inhibitors, ARBs, NSAIDs ⇔ Eplerenone is preferred in patients with gynaecomastia
Urogenital infections due to glycosuria	Contraindications: pregnancy, eGFR <20 ml/min/1.73 m^2 Mild diuretic properties ⇔ Insulin, sulfonylurea

Diuretics and calcium antagonists are more effective in patients of West African or South African descent, because hypertension is more often caused by sodium sensitivity, relatively high plasma volume, and low plasma renin levels.

ADVERSE EFFECTS	NOTES
• Hypotension (risk of falling in the elderly ↑) • Bradycardia • Arrhythmias • Headache • Impotence	Beta blockers belong to the class-II antiarrhythmics that slow AV conduction via the β1 receptors. Sotalol is also a class-III antiarrhythmic. ⇔ Arrhythmias (sotalol): risk ↑ in patients with hypokalaemia (loop and thiazide diuretics, laxatives) and renal impairment (NSAIDs, HF, dehydration) Labetalol and carvedilol also have an alfa-receptor mediated effect Sotalol has specific class III antiarrhythmic properties compared to other beta blockers

Calcium antagonists

	MEDICATION	MECHANISM OF ACTION	INDICATIONS
CALCIUM ANTAGONISTS	**Dihydropyridines** (e.g. amlodipine, nifedipine)	Calcium antagonists block the slow calcium channels (L-type), resulting in vasodilation of the coronary and systemic vasculature	• Hypertension • Stable angina pectoris • Vasospastic angina pectoris • Raynaud's phenomenon
	Non-dihydropiridines (e.g. verapamil, diltiazem)	Increased contractility and decreased conduction in the SA and AV node (class IV antiarrhythmics)	• AF • Angina pectoris • SVT • Symptomatic extrasystoles

Table 52 // Calcium antagonists
AV, atrioventricular; SA, sinoatrial; SVT, supraventricular tachycardia

RAS inhibitors

	MEDICATION	MECHANISM OF ACTION	INDICATIONS
RAS INHIBITORS	**ACE inhibitors** (e.g. captopril, enalapril, lisinopril)	Block RAS by decreasing the conversion of angiotensin I (ATI) to ATII, resulting in vasodilation, glomerular filtration pressure ↓, aldosterone ↓, cardiac hypertrophy ↓ and smooth muscle hypertrophy ↓	• HF • Hypertension • Diabetic nephropathy • Prophylaxis after ACS
	Angiotensin receptor neprilysin inhibitors (ARNI) (e.g. sacubitril-valsartan)	• Sacubitril: blocks the action of neprilysin, preventing breakdown of natriuretic peptides • Valsartan (ARB) inhibits RAS system	• HF • Combination of valsartan/sacubitril in chronic HF with reduced ejection fraction
	ARBs (e.g. losartan, valsartan)	Block ATII receptor type 1 without affecting bradykinin	Alternative to ACE inhibitor for dry cough (or angioedema)

Table 53 // RAS inhibitors
ACE, angiotensin-converting enzyme; ACS, acute coronary syndrome; ARBs, angiotensin receptor blockers; RAS, renin-angiotensin-system

ADVERSE EFFECTS	NOTES
• Hypotension, risk of falling • Reflex tachycardia • Flushing, headache • Peripheral oedema • Constipation	⇔ Combination with beta blockers can lead to HF, hypotension and even an MI in high-risk patients (past MI)
• Headaches, dizziness • Bradycardia, hypotension • AV conduction disorder • Flushing	💡 Do not start in case of HF, 2nd or 3rd-degree AV block, sick sinus syndrome ⇔ Risk of bradycardia, hypotension, conduction disorders or even MI with class II (beta blockers) and class I and III antiarrhythmics (quinidine, amiodarone)

ADVERSE EFFECTS	NOTES
• Orthostatic hypotension (elderly: first-dose hypotension) • Dry cough (bradykinin), angioedema • Renal function ↓, hyperkalaemia	💡 Start low and go slow in elderly patients due to risk of orthostasis ⇔ Risk of renal insufficiency: unilateral/bilateral renal arterial stenosis, dehydration, sepsis, HF, NSAIDs and diuretics ⇔ Risk of hyperkalaemia ↑ in patients with DM, renal failure, HF, ACE inhibitors, ARBs, NSAIDs. Halve dose if serum K^+ >5.5 mmol/L, stop at >6.0.
• Hypotension • Renal function ↓ • Hyperkalaemia	💡 Contraindications: history of angioedema, bilateral renal artery stenosis, pregnancy, eGFR <30 ml/min/1.73 m^2 💡 A washout period of 36h after ACE-I therapy is required to minimise the risk of angioedema ⇔ MRA, potassium suppletion, NSAID, trimethoprim
As an ACE inhibitor; lower risk of dry cough and angioedema	⇔ Risk of hyperkalaemia ↑ in patients with DM, renal failure, HF, ACE inhibitors, ARBs, NSAIDs. Halve dose if serum K^+ >5.5 mmol/L, stop at >6.0. 💡 The combination preparate sacubutril/valsartan improves survival in HF

> **Indications for ACE inhibitors**
> ACE inhibitors are the 1st choice for hypertension at age <50, hypertension with DM (without microalbuminuria), HF or chronic kidney disease (even with microalbuminuria).

> **The paradoxical effect of ACE inhibitors on renal function**
> Although ACE inhibitors improve kidney function in patients with proteinuria, caution is advised in patients with unilateral/bilateral renal arterial stenosis and pre-existing kidney disease, because they further reduce intraglomerular pressure and thus reduce filtration.

Other HF medication

MEDICATION	MECHANISM OF ACTION	INDICATIONS
Vericiguat	Simulation cGMP and soluble guanylate cyclase (sGC) → smooth muscle cell relaxation, hypertrophy ↓, inflammation ↓ and fibrosis ↓	HF with reduced ejection fraction

Table 54 // Other HF medication

Blood glucose-lowering agents

MEDICATION		MECHANISM OF ACTION
BLOOD GLUCOSE-LOWERING AGENT	**Biguanides** (i.e. metformin)	• Inhibits gluconeogenesis in the liver and glycogenolysis in the liver • Increases peripheral insulin sensitivity
	Sulphonylureas (SU) derivatives • Short-acting: tolbutamide, gliclazide • Long-acting: glimepiride	Sulphonylurea derivatives stimulate insulin release through the KATP channels of the pancreas
	Insulin • Short-acting: aspart, lispro • Intermediate-acting: NPH (Humulin N®) • Long-acting: glargine (Lantus®)	There are several types of synthetic insulin, distinguished by their duration of action: short- (4-5h) intermediate- (12-16h) and long-acting (>24h)

Table 55A // Blood glucose-lowering agents

DPP-4, dipeptidyl peptidase 4 inhibitors; GLP-1, glucagon-like peptide 1; KATP channels, ATP-sensitive K^+ channels; SGLT2, sodium-glucose cotransporter 2 inhibitors

Treatment of life-threatening hyperkalaemia
In patients with hyperkalaemia with severe symptoms such as paralysis or ECG abnormalities, administer calcium gluconate to reduce the risk of fatal arrhythmias. Insulin-glucose infusion can then be used to rapidly lower potassium levels. Resonium is a longer-term option for lowering potassium levels.

The five pillars of HF treatment
The five drug categories that should be initiated in every patient with HF are: beta blocker, ACE inhibitor, SGLT2 inhibitor, neprilysin inhibitor, and MRA.

ADVERSE EFFECTS	NOTES
• Hypotension • Anaemia	Risk of cardiovascular mortality and hospitalisations ↓ in patients with HFrEF Contraindication: pregnancy ⇔ Other sGC stimulators, PDE5 inhibitors

ADVERSE EFFECTS	NOTES
• GI disorders (nausea, vomiting, diarrhoea) • Lactate acidosis (accumulation due to reduced renal excretion)	⇔ Risk of lactate acidosis ↓ in cases of diuretics use, alcohol abuse, HF, chronic hypoxaemia (COPD, sepsis) and chronic kidney disease (<30 ml/min/1.73 m²: do not administer; between 30-60 ml/min max. 1000 mg/d)
• Hypoglycaemia (<4 mmol/L; leads to tachycardia, agitation, tremor, sweating and possibly even reduced consciousness), especially with long-acting sulphonylurea derivatives • Weight ↑	⇔ Hypoglycaemia: especially in the elderly, with hepatic or renal insufficiency, excessive exertion, skipping meals and reduced intake. ⊗ Do not give glibenclamide to elderly patients! ⚠ In cases of hypoglycaemia: • Increase carbohydrate or glucose intake • Administer IV glucose or 1 mg glucagon IM or SC in patients with impaired consciousness (glucagon counteracts insulin)
• Hypoglycaemia (see risk factors in the next column; overdose may also occur) • Weight ↑	

MEDICATION		MECHANISM OF ACTION
BLOOD GLUCOSE-LOWERING AGENT	**GLP-1 agonists** (-glutide)	• Activate GLP-1 receptors, stimulate insulin secretion (glucose-dependent) • Suppress glucagon secretion
	DPP-4 inhibitors (-gliptin)	Inhibits the DPP-4 enzyme, so human GLP-1 ↑
	SGLT2 inhibitors (-gliflozin)	• Reversible inhibition of sodium-glucose cotransporter in the tubular system of the kidneys • Increases glucose (and sodium) excretion via urine

Table 55B // Blood glucose-lowering agents

DPP-4, dipeptidyl peptidase 4 inhibitors; GLP-1, glucagon-like peptide 1; KATP channels, ATP-sensitive K^+ channels; SGLT2, sodium-glucose cotransporter 2 inhibitors

Hypoglycaemia unawareness: initial symptoms of hypoglycaemia may be masked by non-selective beta blockers (especially in DM1 and 2 with long-term insulin use). Non-selective beta blockers may also delay glucose level recovery after hypoglycaemia.

In patients with atherosclerotic and non-atherosclerotic cardiovascular disease SGLT2 inhibitors and GLP-1 agonists are the first choice for reducing cardiovascular risk.

TREATMENT	
STEP 1	• Start on metformin 2-3x/d 1 tablet. Adjust dosage according to blood glucose and renal function. • In cardiac patients start SGLT2 inhibitors
STEP 2	Add a sulphonylurea derivative, preferably gliclazide 1x/d 1 controlled release tablet (risk of hypoglycaemia and vascular complications ↓)
STEP 3	Add NPH insulin once daily. Insulin isophane is preferred. Switch to insulin glargine or detemir in cases of nocturnal hypoglycaemia or fluctuating glucose levels. Alternative: DPP4 inhibitor or GLP-1 agonist.
STEP 4	Switch to a multi-dose insulin regimen: choose a 1. Mixed insulin regimen 2x/d, e.g. insulin aspart/aspart protamine, or 2. Add a short-acting insulin 3x/d with meals in addition to an intermediate or long-acting insulin. Note: this increases the risk of hypoglycaemia, so the sulphonylurea derivative must often be discontinued.

Table 56 // Pharmacological treatment for DM type 2

ADVERSE EFFECTS	NOTES
• Gastric emptying ↓ and sensation of satiety ↑ • Lower food intake resulting in weight loss	• No hypoglycaemia due to glucose dependence • GLP-1 agonist initiation can have GI adverse effects. Watch out for dehydration!
• Urogenital infections due to high urinary glucose • Polyuria, pollakisuria	Improves left ventricular function by lowering cardiac pre- and afterload

It is recommended that women with diabetes discontinue all antidiabetic medications prior to pregnancy and start insulin. Insulin use increases risk of hypertension, pre-eclampsia, prematurity, macrosomia, hyperbilirubinaemia, hypocalcaemia, and polycythaemia. Metformin and SU derivates may be considered as an alternative if the benefits outweigh the risks.

Cardiac glycosides

Digoxin is the only cardiac glycoside that is still prescribed. Cardiac glycosides inhibit Na^+-K^+-ATPase in the cardiomyocyte cell membrane. More sodium therefore remains in the cell, which can be exchanged for calcium during each contraction. This has the following effects:

1. Heart contractility ↑ (positive inotropy)
2. Heart rate ↓ (negative chronotropy)
3. AV conduction ↓ (negative dromotropy)

INDICATIONS	ADVERSE EFFECTS	NOTES
• AF/SVT with rapid ventricular response (rhythm control) • AF in chronic HF with systolic dysfunction	• Conduction disorders or arrhythmias (risk in hypokalaemia and renal impairment ↑) • Bradycardia • Dizziness, vision disorders • Watch out for digitalis poisoning!	• Digoxin has a narrow therapeutic index (0.8-2.0 ng/ml), posing a risk of digitalis poisoning (nausea, vomiting, vision disorders and arrhythmias) • Lower dose in the elderly and patients with impaired renal function and thyroid function

Table 57 // Digoxin

Lipid-lowering agents

MEDICATION	MECHANISM OF ACTION	INDICATIONS
Bempedoic acid	Inhibition of adenosine triphosphate citrate lyase (enzyme upstream of HMG-CoA reductase)	• Hypercholesterolaemia • Mixed dyslipidaemia • Statin intolerance
Bezafibrate, gemfibrozil	Fibrates inhibit VLDL synthesis in the liver and stimulate VLDL degradation, with a strong effect on TG ↓ and a mild effect on cholesterol ↓ and HDL ↑	• Severe hypertriglyceridemia • If there is statin intolerance: - Primary hypercholesterolaemia - Mixed hyperlipidaemia - Secondary CVD prevention
Cholestyramine, colesevelam	Synthetic bile acid sequestrant that interrupts enterohepatic circulation of bile acids, with cholesterol synthesis ↑ → LDL ↓	• Combined with a statin in patients with primary hypercholesterolaemia or for secondary CVD prevention (10-year risk >20% and LDL target value not achieved), or in patients with a statin intolerance • Itching due to bile duct obstruction (bile-acid-binding resin)
Ezetimibe	Inhibits cholesterol absorption in the small intestine, with total cholesterol ↓, LDL ↓, TG ↓ and HDL ↑	
Proprotein convertase subtilisin/kexin type 9 (PCSK-9) inhibitors (e.g. evolocumab, alirocumab)	Degradation of LDL-receptor ↓ → hepatic LDL-R expression ↑ → plasma LDL-C levels ↓	• Familial hypercholesterolaemia • Persistent high LDL despite statin and ezetimibe • Statine intolerance
Statins (e.g. simvastatin, atorvastatin, rosuvastatin)	Inhibition of cholesterol biosynthesis via the HMG-CoA reductase enzyme, with total cholesterol ↓, LDL ↓ and to a lesser extent TG ↓. They also have a positive effect on endothelial function, plaque stability and thrombus formation.	• Prevention in patients with atherosclerotic cardiovascular disease or DM • Familial hypercholesterolaemia • Primary hypercholesterolaemia • Mixed dyslipidaemia

Table 58 // Lipid-lowering agents
CVD, cardiovascular disease; HDL, high-density lipoprotein; IgG1, immunoglobulin G type 1; LDL, low density lipoprotein; PCSK9, proprotein convertase subtilisin/kexin type 9; VLDL, very low-density lipoprotein

ADVERSE EFFECTS	NOTES
• Serum transaminases ↑, creatinine, and uric acid • Gout	💡 Primary activation in liver avoiding possible myotoxicity associated with statin therapy. Can therefore be used in statin intolerant patients.
• Dyspepsia, abdominal pain, diarrhoea • Headache, rare muscle pain • Impaired liver function, hepatitis, cholelithiasis (check liver function)	⇔ Risk of myopathy (rhabdomyolysis) when used concomitantly with statins ↑
• Constipation, flatulence • Dyspepsia and nausea • Resorption of VKA, digoxin, levothyroxine, tetracyclines ↓	💡 The adverse effects and interaction profile of colesevelam and ezetimibe are more favourable than that of cholestyramine
• Abdominal pain, diarrhoea, flatulence • Combined with statin: headache, muscle pain, rhabdomyolysis	
• Local injection site rejection • Hypersensitivity • Upper respiratory tract infection • Myalgia, arthralgia	💡 Monoclonal antibody 💡 Lp(a) reduction of ± 30-40%
• Muscle pain, muscle cramps • Rare myopathy (1-7%), liver disease or rhabdomyolysis (possibly with acute renal insufficiency due to myoglobinaemia) • Hyperglycaemia (more common with atorvastatin and rosuvastatin)	⇔ Risk of myopathy and rhabdomyolysis ↑ with CYP3A4 inhibitors (oral antimycotics, HIV protease inhibitors, grapefruit juice, ciclosporin, verapamil, diltiazem) and concomitant use of fibrates or ezetimibe

Benzodiazepines

	MEDICATION	MECHANISM OF ACTION
BENZODIAZEPINES	**Midazolam** (ultra-short)	• Benzodiazepines enhance the inhibitory effect of the neurotransmitter GABA, with hypnotic, anxiolytic, anticonvulsant and muscle-relaxant effects • The main differences between the agents are their respective elimination half-lives ($t_{1/2}$=2-3.5h/2-4h/5h/7-11h/4-15h/20-48h, respectively) • Oxazepam is the active metabolite of diazepam • Zolpidem is a benzodiazepine-like hypnotic, which acts rapidly ($t_{1/2}$ 2-4h) and briefly, and mainly has a sedative effect in low doses
	Zolpidem (ultra-short)	
	Zopiclon (short)	
	Temazepam (short)	
	Oxazepam (short)	
	Diazepam (long)	
	Lorazepam	

Table 59 // Benzodiazepines
GABA, gamma-aminobutyric acid; OSAS, obstructive sleep apnea syndrome

INDICATION (CORRELATION WITH $T_{1/2}$)	MIDA-ZOLAM	ZOLPI-DEM	ZOPI-CLON	TEMAZE-PAM	OXAZE-PAM	DIAZE-PAM	LORAZE-PAM
Sleep disorders	X	X	X	X			X
Anxiety disorders: social phobia/ generalised					X	X	X
Alcohol abstinence					X	X	X
Epileptic seizure/ febrile convulsion/ delirium	X					X	X

Table 60 // Indications of benzodiazepines

To prevent tolerance and dependence, it is recommended that benzodiazepines be prescribed for <2 wk and up to 4 wk. It is recommended to prescribe benzodiazepines as a sleep aid only after other non-pharmacological options have been unsuccessful (e.g. sleep hygiene, cognitive behavioural therapy).

If a patient develops tolerance and dependence despite taking precautions, the risk of rebound symptoms can be reduced by slowly tapering off and switching to a long-acting benzodiazepine.

ADVERSE EFFECTS	NOTES
• Drowsiness, alertness ↓ (watch out when driving!) • Muscle weakness (risk of falling) • Anterograde amnesia • Tolerance and dependence • Rebound phenomenon following abstinence (anxiety, sleep problems) • Paradoxical reaction • Respiratory depression	⇔ Risk of adverse effects ↑ in the elderly (greater fat mass/volume of distribution) and patients using alcohol, recreational drugs, opioids and psychotropics (antipsychotics, antidepressants) ⇔ Respiratory depression: COPD and OSAS ⇔ Paradoxical reaction: especially in children ▲ In case of overdose (respiratory depression), administer IV flumazenil, a short-acting (!) benzodiazepine antagonist

For the latest information about doses, adverse effects, and more:

- United Kingdom: *www.medicines.org.uk/emc*
- Canada: *go.drugbank.com*
- Netherlands: *www.farmacotherapeutischkompas.nl*

Antiseizure medication

Medication tapering is preferred for women who are actively looking to conceive and patients who have been in remission for >2y.

Lamotrigine and levetiracetam are the first-choice maintenance therapies for women of childbearing age, preferably as monotherapy at the lowest effective dose.
Carbamazepine, phenytoin, and valproate are known to be teratogenic. Valproate has been shown to carry the highest risk of major congenital malformations. Therefore, these agents should not be prescribed to women of childbearing age.

In case of **brain tumour-related epilepsy (BTRE)**, the use of levetiracetam, lacosamide, or valproic acid have been proven effective. If levetiracetam is ineffective, lacosamide and valproic acid can also be used as add-on medication.

	MEDICATION	MECHANISM OF ACTION	INDICATIONS
ANTISEIZURE MEDICATION	**Barbiturates** (phenobarbital, primidone)	• GABA agonist • Primidone is converted to phenobarbital in the body	• Generalised and focal epilepsy • Status epilepticus • Off-label 1st choice for neonatal convulsions
	Valproic acid	• Exact mechanism of action unknown • GABA concentration ↑ (likely) and sodium and potassium channel sensitivity ↓	• Maintenance therapy generalised and focal epilepsy • Status epilepticus (high-dose IV)
	Phenytoin	• Exact mechanism of action in epilepsy unknown • Improves AV conduction by suppressing spontaneous depolarisation of atrial and ventricular tissue	• Maintenance therapy focal epilepsy or tonic-clonic seizures in generalised epilepsy • Status epilepticus (high-dose IV)
	Levetiracetam	• Exact mechanism of action unknown • Influence on intraneuronal calcium level, GABA and glycine channel sensitivity, interaction with SVA2	• Monotherapy for focal epilepsy, with or without secondary generalisation (age >16) • Monotherapy for generalised epilepsy • Adjuvant therapy for focal epilepsy (age >1 mo), myoclonic seizures in juvenile myoclonic epilepsy (age >12 y) and primary generalised tonic-clonic seizures in idiopathic generalised epilepsy (age >12 y) • Status epilepticus (high-dose IV)

Table 61 // Antiseizure medication

AV, atrioventricular; ECG, electrocardiogram; GABA, gamma-aminobutyric acid; PCOS, polycystic ovary syndrome; SVA2, synaptic vesicle protein 2; UGT, uridinedifosfaat-glucuronosyl-transferase

Elderly patients generally metabolise antiseizure medication at a slower rate and are therefore more susceptible to dose-related adverse effects.

Many antiseizure medication have a major effect on driving ability.

ADVERSE EFFECTS	NOTES
• Fatigue, lethargy, headache, dizziness, vomiting, nausea, ataxia, nystagmus, diplopia, acute psychotic reactions • Cardiorespiratory depression • Idiosyncratic: rash	⇔ CYP3A induction ⇔ Concentration ↑ due to valproic acid
• Tremor, nausea, sedation, parkinsonism, hair loss, amenorrhoea, risk of neural tube defect in foetus ↑, risk of PCOS ↑ • Idiosyncratic: hepatotoxicity, pancreatitis	⇔ CYP2C9 ↓, Pgp ↑ ⇔ Plasma phenytoin level ↓, enhanced action of barbiturates ⇔ Teratogenic
• Nausea, constipation, dizziness, ataxia, nystagmus, tremor/dyskinesia, confusion, speech disorder, apathy, neuropathy, visual disturbances, arrhyth-mia, effect on oestrogen metabolism (oral contraceptives clearance ↑) • Idiosyncratic: gum hyperplasia, rash	⇔ CI: generalised tonic-clonic seizures with myoclonuses or absences: risk of counter-productive effect ⇔ Strong CYP3A4 inducer ⇔ Blood level in conjunction with carbamazepine ↓, with e.g. alcohol consumption ↑ ⇔ Teratogenic ⊗ CYP2C9 polymorphism: manifested as noticeably more or more severe adverse effects 💡 IV administration only with continuous ECG and respiratory monitoring because of risk of hypotensia, arrhythmias, and CNS depression 💡 Measure free fraction in case of hypoalbuminuria and watch for displacement of albumin by valproic acid
• Nasopharyngitis, headache, drowsiness, ataxia, sedation • Idiosyncratic: rash	💡 Dosage should be adjusted to renal function

💡 Testing serum concentrations of antiseizure medication is useful in case of treatment with phenytoin, use of multiple antiseizure medication, dose-related adverse effects, suspicion of noncompliance, possible interactions, dialysis and during pregnancy.

💡 Because many antiseizure medication induce the CYP mechanism, close attention must be paid to how different antiseizure medication can lower or raise each other's levels when prescribed together.

Antibiotics

	MEDICATION	MECHANISM OF ACTION	COVERAGE
ANTIBIOTICS (AB)	**Penicillins** • Penicillinase-resistant (e.g. flucloxacillin) • Broad-spectrum (e.g. amoxicillin, piperacillin)	The three groups of beta-lactam antibiotics inhibit the synthesis of bacterial cell wall peptidoglycan and derive their names from their characteristic beta-lactam ring. In combination with a beta-lactamase inhibitor such as clavulanic acid or tazobactam, they can also be used to treat beta-lactamase-forming bacteria.	• Predominantly active against G+ pathogens; flucloxacillin and augmentin are also active against beta-lactamase-producing pathogens, such as *Staphylococcus aureus* • Broad-spectrum: also active against some G- bacteria
	Cephalosporins • 1st generation: e.g. cefazolin • 2nd generation: e.g. cefuroxime • 3rd generation: e.g. ceftazidime • 4th generation: e.g. cefepime		• Cefazolin: narrow spectrum (G+) • Cefuroxime: more active against G- pathogens (beta-lactamase insensitivity) • Ceftazidime: broader spectrum, especially effective against G- bacteria
	Carbapenems (e.g. meropenem)		Very broad-spectrum AB used primarily to treat highly resistant G- bacteria, e.g. ESBL
	Quinolones (e.g. ciprofloxacin, levofloxacin)	Inhibition of DNA transcription and replication by inhibiting DNA gyrase	• Broad spectrum (especially active against G- (enterocolic) bacteria, also *Haemophilus influenzae*, *Campylobacter* and *Pseudomonas*) • Ciprofloxacin is the 1st choice for treating complicated UTIs. High oral availability.
	Aminoglycosides (e.g. gentamicin)	Block the initiation of protein synthesis	• Mainly active against aerobic G- rods, as well as various G+ organisms • Synergy with beta-lactam antibiotics
	Macrolides (e.g. azithromycin, clarithromycin)	Bacteriostatic action through protein synthesis inhibition	Similar to penicillins, but with a broader spectrum (*Mycoplasma pneumoniae*, *Legionella pneumophila*, *Mycobacterium avium*); use in cases of penicillin resistance/ sensitivity.

Table 62A // Antibiotics
AB, antibiotics; ESBL, extended spectrum beta-lactamase; G+, gram-positive; G-, gram-negative; UTIs, urinary tract infections

ADVERSE EFFECTS	NOTES
• GI: nausea, abdominal pain, diarrhoea • Toxicodermies (7-8% with amoxicillin) • Hypersensitivity (1%) • Anaphylactic shock (0.01-0.04%)	⇔ There is cross-sensitivity between different types of penicillins. Cross-sensitivity with cephalosporins is much less common. 💡 Risk of pseudomembranous colitis (*Clostridium difficile*)
• GI: nausea, abdominal pain, diarrhoea • Bone marrow depression (thrombocytopenia, leukopenia, granulocytopenia) • Haemolytic anaemia	⇔ Cross-sensitivity with penicillins (10-15%) ⇔ No simultaneous parenteral administration with solutions containing calcium → precipitation
• GI: nausea, abdominal pain, diarrhoea • Bone marrow depression (thrombocytopenia, leukopenia, granulocytopenia) • Haemolytic anaemia	⇔ Concomitant use of bacteriostatic AB → bactericidal activity of carbapenems ↓ (also applies to other beta-lactam ABs)
• GI: nausea, abdominal pain, diarrhoea • Hypersensitivity • Achilles tendon rupture (with prolonged use)	⇔ Complex formation with calcium, magnesium, zinc, iron → strong absorption ↓ (antacids, milk, iron preparations)
• Ototoxicity (vertigo, ataxia, deafness; irreversible) • Nephrotoxicity (reversible)	⇔ Ototoxicity: risk ↑ with loop diuretics ⇔ Nephrotoxicity: risk ↑ in renal insufficiency 💡 Therapeutic drug monitoring necessary when administering repeated doses due to narrow therapeutic index
• GI: nausea, abdominal pain, diarrhoea • Hypersensitivity	⇔ Macrolides are potent CYP3A4 inhibitors (increased risk of adverse effects when used concomitantly with statins, e.g. myopathy and rhabdomyolysis) 💡 Risk of QT prolongation ↑

💡 Antibiotic resistancy can be region or even hospital-specific. Always check your local antibiotic protocol for the first choice antibiotic in specific situations.

	MEDICATION	MECHANISM OF ACTION	COVERAGE
ANTIBIOTICS (AB)	**Tetracyclines** (e.g. doxycycline, tetracycline)	Bacteriostatic action due to protein synthesis inhibition	Very broad spectrum, covering *Mycoplasma, Rickettsia, Chlamydia, Borrelia*, spirochetes and protozoa
	Sulfonamides (e.g. cotrimoxazole: sulfonamide + trimethoprim)	Synergistic inhibition of folate synthesis and therefore of bacterial DNA/RNA	Most G+ and G- microorganisms, as well as *Pneumocystis jirovecii* (pneumonia in HIV) and *Toxoplasma gondii* (toxoplasmosis)

Table 62B // Antibiotics

Causes of lack of response to treatment: resistance, pathogen falls outside AB spectrum, non-infectious underlying cause (e.g. autoimmune disease, malignancy or drug fever), focus of infection is not/hardly reached (e.g. abscess, empyema, prosthesis/catheter), poor local circulation (DM, peripheral vascular disease).

ANTIBIOTIC	GRAM-POSITIVE						
	Cocci						Anaerobic
	MRSA	*Staphylococcus epidermidis*	MMSA	*Enterococcus faecium*	*Enterococcus faecalis*	*Streptococcus*	*Clostridium, Peptostreptococcus*
Amoxicillin			■	■	■	■	
Azithromycin							
Cefazolin			■			■	
Cefepime			■			■	■
Ceftazidime							
Ceftriaxone			■			■	■
Cefuroxime			■			■	■
Clavulanic acid			■	■	■	■	■
Clindamycin	■		■			■	■
Cotrimoxazole	■	■	■		■	■	■

Table 63A // Antibiotic spectrum of activity
Please note that this is a general table, local protocols and resistance may vary

ADVERSE EFFECTS	NOTES
• Photosensitivity (photodermatitis, photoonycholysis) • Calcium chelation: dental discoloration, dental hypoplasia and delayed osteogenesis	Chelation of metal ions: see Quinolones Tooth discoloration/reduced osteogenesis: do not prescribe for pregnant women from week 16 or for children younger than age 8 ⇔ Enhanced action of oral anticoagulants
• GI: nausea, abdominal pain, diarrhoea • Hypersensitivity • Bone marrow suppression	⇔ Methotrexate potentiates bone marrow suppression, HIV is a risk factor ⇔ Via CYP2C9 inhibition → VKA action ↑ (risk of bleeding and INR elevation)

Bridging and switch therapy
As soon as the pathogen and sensitivity pattern are known, a narrower, more targeted treatment should be chosen to replace the initial broad-spectrum therapy (lower risk of resistance, less impact on endogenous flora and fewer adverse effects). If the patient's clinical status improves, it is also important to switch from IV AB to oral AB after 2-3d, or after 3-4d for more severe infections.

GRAM-NEGATIVE									
Anaerobic	**Cocci/coccobacilli**			**Bacilli**					
Bacteroides, Fusobacterium	***Nesseria meningitidis***	***Haemophilus influenzae***	***Moraxella***	***Escherichia coli***	***Klebsiella pneumoniae***	***Proteus, Mirabilis***	***Pseudomonas***	**ESCAPPM* organisms**	***Legionella***
		■							
									■
	■	■		■	■	■			
■	■	■	■	■	■	■	■	■	
		■	■	■	■	■	■		
	■	■	■	■	■	■			
	■	■	■	■	■	■			
■	■	■	■	■	■	■			
■									
■	■	■	■	■	■	■			■

ANTIBIOTIC	GRAM-POSITIVE						
	Cocci						Anaerobic
	MRSA	*Staphylococcus epidermidis*	MMSA	*Enterococcus faecium*	*Enterococcus faecalis*	*Streptococcus*	*Clostridium, Peptostreptococcus*
Daptomycin	■	■	■	■	■	■	
Ertapenem		■	■			■	■
Erythromycin							
Flucloxacillin		■	■			■	
Fusidic acid	■	■	■		■		
Gentamicin	■		■	■	■		
Imipenem		■	■		■	■	■
Linezolid	■	■	■	■	■	■	
Meropenem		■	■			■	■
Metronidazole							■
Moxifloxacin		■	■		■	■	■
Penicillin				■	■	■	
Piperacillin			■		■	■	■
Rifampicin	■	■	■				
Tazobactam			■		■	■	■
Teicoplanin	■	■	■	■	■	■	
Ticarcillin			■	■	■	■	■
Tigecycline	■	■	■	■	■	■	■
Tobramycin					■		
Trimethoprim				■			
Vancomycin	■	■	■	■	■	■	

Table 63B // Antibiotic spectrum of activity
Please note that this is a general table, local protocols and resistance may vary

GRAM-NEGATIVE									
Anaerobic	**Cocci/coccobacilli**			**Bacilli**					
Bacteroides, Fusobacterium	***Nesseria meningitidis***	***Haemophilus influenzae***	***Moraxella***	***Escherichia coli***	***Klebsiella pneumoniae***	***Proteus, Mirabilis***	***Pseudomonas***	**ESCAPPM* organisms**	***Legionella***
■	■	■	■	■	■	■		■	
									■
	■	■							
				■	■	■	■	■	
■	■	■	■	■	■	■	■	■	
■	■	■	■	■	■	■	■	■	
■									
■	■	■	■	■	■	■		■	■
	■								
■	■	■	■	■	■	■			
	■	■							
■	■	■	■	■	■	■			
■	■	■	■	■	■	■	■		
■	■		■	■	■			■	■
				■	■	■	■	■	
				■	■				■

ESCAPPM is a mnemonic for organisms with inducible beta-lactamase activity. These organisms are ***E****nterocacter spp.*, ***C****itrobacter freundii*, ***A****eromonas spp.*, ***P****roteus spp.* (excluding *P. mirabilis*), ***P****rovidencia spp.* and ***M****organella morganii*.

IV fluids policy

Many patients who are hospitalised will have an infusion. An infusion is a prescribed medication, just like antibiotics and analgesics. In fact, the infusion is the most frequently administered medicine in our daily care. In this section, we discuss the required basic knowledge about infusion fluids and their distribution throughout the body and we will offer practical tips for the formulation of a suitable IV fluids policy.

Body water

The human body consists of about 50 to 70 percent water. The "Total Body Water" (TBW) depends on the body composition and on gender and age. Adult men consist of about 60 percent water and adult women and the elderly consist of about 50 percent water. Obese individuals also have relatively less body water. The body water is distributed over various compartments (see Table 64).

TOTAL BODY WATER TBW = 42L (based on an adult man weighing 70 kg)		
Intracellular compartment 25L (60% TBW)	**Extracellular compartment** 17L (40% TBW)	
	Extravascular (interstitium) 14L (33% TBW)	**Intravascular (plasma)** 3L (7% TBW)

Table 64 // Distribution of fluids in the human body, for a man weighing 70 kg. TBW = Total Body Water

Any IV fluids that are administered will initially form part of the plasma (intravascular) compartment. If the fluid with dissolved substances passes the capillary wall, then a proportion of the fluid will move to the interstitium. The plasma and interstitium together form the extracellular compartment. If the fluid crosses the cell membrane thereafter, the fluid will reach the intracellular compartment. The capillary membrane is readily permeable to water and electrolytes, but not to proteins (under physiological circumstances). The cell membrane is readily permeable to water, but not to electrolytes and proteins. Therefore, both membranes are semi-permeable.

Plasma volume is not the same as **blood volume**. Blood consists of plasma (water with dissolved substances) and cells. The plasma volume is responsible for the clinical presentations of hypovolaemia and fluid overload.

In clinical practice, when someone refers to loss of fluid in the **third space**, this refers to extracellular fluid accumulation such as pleural effusion and ascites.

Osmotic and hydrostatic pressure

The fluid distribution between compartments is determined by the osmotic and hydrostatic pressure. Osmosis of water across a semi-permeable membrane takes place if the two compartments have different osmotic potential and always proceeds from the compartment with a low osmotic potential (= low concentration of dissolved substances) to the compartment with a high osmotic potential (= high concentration of dissolved substances, see Figure 17). The distribution between the intracellular and extracellular compartment is determined by the difference in osmolality: the total amount of small dissolved substances (including Na^+, K^+, urea, and glucose) per kg fluid.

The terms "osmolarity" and "osmolality" are sometimes used interchangeably. Although these values are virtually identical for plasma, these terms do not refer to the same concept. The term **osmolarity** refers to the number of dissolved particles **per litre**. The term **osmolality** refers to the number of dissolved particles **per kilogram**.

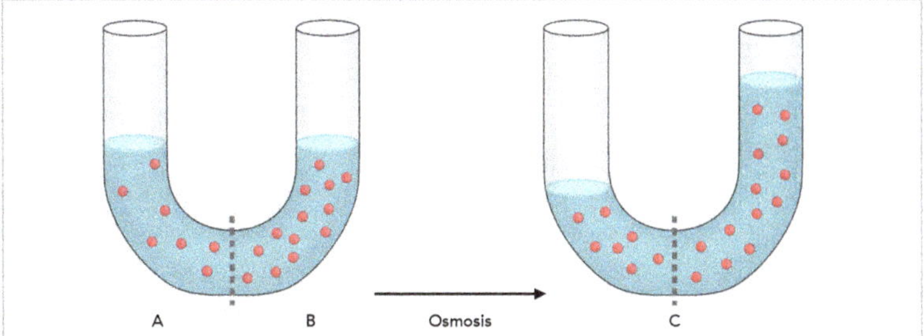

Figure 17 // Osmosis

A: Relatively low concentration of particles **B:** Relatively high concentration of particles **C:** Same concentration of particles

Within the extracellular compartment, the hydrostatic and colloid osmotic pressure determine the water distribution between the intravascular and extravascular compartment. The colloid osmotic pressure is determined by proteins that are unable to diffuse out of the blood vessel. The hydrostatic pressure is the pressure exerted by the fluid on the blood vessel wall. Both pressures determine whether or not an administered fluid remains in the circulation.

Oedema (diffusion of fluid from the circulation) is caused by a decrease in colloid osmotic pressure (e.g. with hypoalbuminaemia) and/or an increase in the hydrostatic venous pressure (e.g. with HF). In addition, decreased removal of interstitial fluid can also play a role (e.g. with lymphatic obstruction).

Characteristics of infusion fluids

Crystalloids are the most commonly used infusion fluids and are subdivided into hypertonic, isotonic and hypotonic fluids. Hypertonic IV fluids (e.g. NaCl 3%) have a higher osmotic potential than the extracellular compartment and cause withdrawal of fluid in the intracellular compartment. As a result, the volume load for the patient will be greater than the original volume that was administered. Isotonic fluids (e.g. NaCl 0.9% and Ringer's lactate) have the same osmotic potential as the extracellular compartment and will therefore not cause any fluid shift between the extracellular and intracellular compartment. However, the composition of these fluids does differ from the composition of the extracellular compartment and can induce hypernatraemia and hyperchloraemia. Hypotonic IV fluids (e.g. glucose 5%, refer below for further explanation) have a lower osmotic potential than the extracellular compartment, meaning that the fluid will readily diffuse from the extracellular to the intracellular compartment. This is due to the fact that intravenously administered glucose will be metabolised and converted to CO_2 and H_2O. The water that is formed will disperse evenly over the intracellular and extracellular compartments. Therefore, administering a glucose 5% solution can be considered the same as giving water (see Figure 18). Hypotonic fluids cause cells to swell, resulting in oedema and potentially even lethal cerebral oedema. Lastly, colloid IV fluids (e.g. hydroxyethyl cellulose) contain large molecules that do not diffuse across the capillary membrane at all, or with great difficulty. They are rarely used in modern IV fluids policy due to equal effects of crystalloids in patients with shock. Some colloids are associated with kidney damage (Hydroxyethyl starch (HES) and dextran). The half-life of infusion fluids like crystalloids is 20 to 40 minutes in healthy patients, but might extend to 80 minutes or longer in the presence of stress, dehydration etc. The half-life of colloids is two to three hours.

See Table 65 for an overview of the indication areas for the IV fluids mentioned in this section.

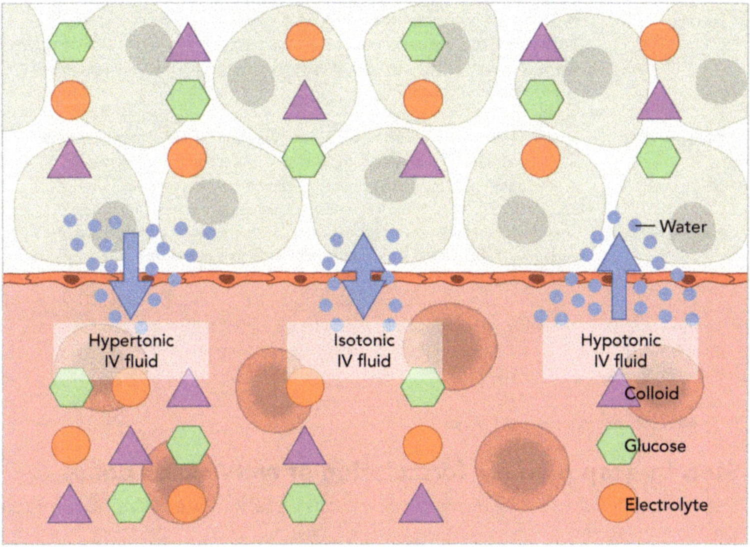

Figure 18 // Effect of hypertonic, isotonic, and hypotonic IV fluids

Crystalloids are generally the first choice for resuscitation fluids.

In the case of clinical signs of shock, a "fluid challenge" is indicated in many cases. Balanced electrolyte solutions are preferred (e.g., Ringer's, Jonisteril). Sodium chloride (NaCl) 0.9% can be used when balanced electrolyte solutions are not available, but NaCl 0.9% is less favourable due to a higher risk of complications (hypernatraemia). In patients with reduced cardiac function (EF <40%), IV fluids should not be administered too quickly due to the inotropic challenges to the heart, though the volume itself will not be an issue.

TYPE OF IV FLUID	INDICATIONS
NaCl 0.9%	• Dehydration (esp. when vomiting, to compensate for loss of Cl) • Hypotension • For certain types of hyponatraemia (an Internal Medicine consultation is recommended in these cases)
Ringer's lactate	Ringer's lactate is often a better choice than NaCl 0.9% in situations requiring large quantities of intravascular filling (e.g. with sepsis), or as a maintenance infusion because it is a balanced, isotonic fluid. Ringer's lactate results in comparable intravascular filling, but less disruption of electrolytes than administration of large volumes of NaCl 0.9%.
Glucose 5%	• Loss of water, evidenced by hyperosmolarity and subsequent hypernatraemia • For overcorrection of hyponatraemia (if contra-correction is indicated) • Peri-operatively for diabetic patients, combined with IV insulin
NaCl 3%	Treatment of symptomatic hyponatraemia. Watch out for a rapid increase in serum sodium or fluid overload (an Internal Medicine consultation is recommended in these cases).
Sodium bicarbonate 1.4% or 8.4%	• Pre-hydration and post-hydration for the administration of IV contrast agents as part of interventions/diagnostic examinations • Hyperkalaemia

Table 65 // Indications for various IV fluids

Step-by-step plan for formulation of an IV fluids policy

The correct IV fluids policy depends on various patient-related factors (see Table 66).

The risk of **phlebitis** should not be taken lightly. It would not be the first time that this is the cause of a *Staphylococcus aureus* bacteraemia. Do not leave a cannula in any longer than strictly necessary and remove the cannula at the first signs of suspected phlebitis.

The quantity of salt in one litre of NaCl 0.9% (9 grams) far exceeds the recommended daily **salt intake**. The recommended salt intake is even lower for patients with HF or kidney failure. Patients with renal function impairment and/or cardiac issues (in short, many elderly patients) are therefore at risk of fluid overload. Therefore, opt for a balanced, isotonic IV fluid as the basic infusion liquid.

STEP	TREATMENT CONSIDERATIONS
1 **Is the patient unstable or dehydrated?**	• You should administer NaCl 0.9% or Ringer's lactate to achieve good intravascular filling, whilst monitoring BP and urine production (target diuresis of at least 0.5 mL/kg/h) • The administration of repeated fluid challenges is the preferred option for unstable patients • Blood products are the preferred option in the case of severe bleeding and haemodynamic instability, but crystalloids can be considered in addition to this • For hyponatraemia or hypernatraemia: considering consulting Internal Medicine
2 **Assess the patient's output (diuresis + other losses)**	• Diuresis (target diuresis of at least 0.5 mL/kg/h). The composition of the urine depends on the circulating volume and use of medication (e.g. diuretics). Replace what the patient has lost • Insensible perspiration ("invisible" loss of fluid via the skin and respiration, depends primarily on (body) temperature and will be higher in the case of a fever). Via the skin (perspiration): more salt than water. Via the respiration: pure water • Gastro-intestinal losses (vomiting, diarrhoea). The patient is losing isotonic electrolyte fluids, so you should supplement with an isotonic fluid. • Other loss via drains, fistulas and NG tubes: refer to section on gastro-intestinal loss • Sequestration of fluid in ascites or other oedemas: colloids, in particular albumin, in patients with ascites or nephrotic syndrome
3 **Determine the patient's own intake**	If you expect that the patient will be able to drink enough (extra) liquids himself, then you should preferably encourage this intake. An IV line restricts the patient's ability to move around and can result in various complications, with phlebitis being the most common complication.
4 **Determine whether any other deficiencies need to be supplemented**	For example, does the patient require extra potassium via the infusion?
5 **Determine whether there are any exceptional circumstances that would require you to opt for a special type of infusion**	An example of this would be a perioperative diabetic patient who requires an insulin/glucose infusion. Observe the relevant guidelines in your centre when prescribing such an infusion.

Table 66 // Step-by-step plan for formulation of an IV fluids policy

A target of 30 mL/kg/24h is generally used to determine the volume of maintenance IV for a patient who is NPO. This number is based on the assumption of an ideal body mass (height in cm - 100). For example, a man who is 180 cm tall should receive a maintenance infusion of approx. 2400 mL Ringer's lactate per 24h. This infusion can be reduced as the patient's intake increases. The infusion should be increased if more fluids are lost. Infusion volumes of more than three litres or less than one litre per 24h are uncommon for maintenance infusions.

Blood transfusion

A blood transfusion is indicated for patients who present with clinically significant bleeding. In such situations, the administration of blood transfusions is preferable to the administration of large volumes of crystalloids. Large volumes of crystalloids will result in dilution of the blood, resulting in a deterioration in blood clotting and a reduction in body temperature. Aim to maintain a Hb above 8.0 g/dL or 5.0 mmol/L. Follow your hospital guidelines. In anaemic, non-bleeding adult patients, including ICU patients, use a restrictive transfusion threshold of 7.0 g/dL or 4.3 mmol/L. In patients with Acute Coronary Syndrome (ACS), undergoing orthopaedic or cardiac surgery the threshold is 8.0 g/dL or 5.0 mmol/L. Do not transfuse more than one unit at a time.

With the exception of administering "uncrossmatched" blood (O^-) for life-threatening bleeding, the blood group and rhesus factor of the donor and recipient should be determined prior to administration of a blood transfusion. Antibody screening and serological cross-matching are also performed when transfusion PRBCs (erythrocytes). A blood transfusion with an incompatible blood group can result in severe, potentially lethal haemolysis (See section *Conditions, Transfusion Reaction*).

- Blood group O^- can be given to anyone in an emergency. Erythrocytes from a donor with blood group O^- do not carry any antigens on their surface, meaning that they will not provoke a reaction in the recipient.
- A person with blood group AB^+ can receive blood from any donor. Blood group AB^+ has both A and B antigens on the surface of the erythrocytes and does not produce any antibodies.

Each unit of PRBCs should result in an increase of Hb by 0.5-0.6 mmol/L.

A low blood pressure is sometimes accepted for patients with significant active blood loss ("permissive hypotension"). Examples of such situations include patients with oesophageal varices, an AAAA or blood loss resulting from traumatic injuries. Maintaining a lower target value ensures that further blood loss is limited, whilst ensuring that perfusion of the vital organs is maintained. Discuss this consideration with your supervisor if you think that your patient may be eligible for this approach.

Management of a patient with...

Clinical reasoning is often described as a continuous interplay between two processes: **pattern recognition** and **hypothetical-deductive reasoning**. Pattern recognition is fast, intuitive and often completely subconscious. The healthcare provider formulates a working diagnosis based on observed similarities to previous cases, in which alternatives are often only briefly considered. If the clinical presentation does not fit a certain pattern, the healthcare provider relies on a slower, more analytical process: hypothetical-deductive reasoning. The healthcare provider consciously considers possible alternative diagnoses, before formulating the final diagnosis. The more experience a person has, the more they can rely on pattern recognition. Conversely, this also means that a young junior doctor at the start of their career will use the slower, hypothetical-deductive reasoning more often, which can be quite tricky during a busy shift. In this section, we offer you guidelines for approaching patients with varying symptoms, so that you can act decisively in situations where you lack the required experience.

Reading guide

- Each diagram starts with a **symptom**, followed by a **differential diagnosis**.
- The diagram then splits into two paths; the left-hand path is for patients assigned to you via an **external route** (e.g. via their GP), the right-hand path is for patients who have already been admitted and assigned to you via an **internal route** (e.g. via the ward nurse).
- After gauging the **urgency** (low/high) over the telephone, you should give the nurse involved in the patient's care **instructions** for the initial care, adapted according to the patient's location. This allows the nurse to get to work, whilst waiting for an assessment by the doctor.
- Each diagram ends with **recommendations for the assessment**.
- Specific treatment instructions are provided in the section *Conditions*.

Local protocols are the main guidelines for your actions. When you are settling into your new job, use this section when discussing cases with your supervisor and your fellow junior doctors. Use the notes section to record any points of attention for your specific context. There is space at the end of the section where you can work out extra symptoms.

When you are contacted about a patient, check the registration system to verify the patient's name and date of birth (and also the patient number). Also record the contact details of the person who called you, so that you can contact him/her at a later stage if necessary.

Often the circumstances for caring for a critically ill patient on a nursing ward are less than ideal. Create some space and calm surroundings to structure the process: ask two nurses to be present in the room (one assisting and one circulating), ensure that you have adequate lighting, move the bedside tables to the bathroom, in very urgent situations any other patients staying in the same room should be moved elsewhere on the ward and the Computer on Wheels (COW) should be moved to the room for immediate access to the patient's details.

You should only implement definitive treatment orders in consultation with your supervisor, unless you have reached another agreement with your supervisor. You should always contact your supervisor if you have any doubts.

Do not hesitate to call your supervisor if you need help.

Diagram 7 // Management of a patient with abdominal pain

The management of a patient with abdominal pain

↓

Consider at least the following

Intra-abdominal

- Gastrointestinal: appendicitis, cholecystitis, cholecystolithiasis, choledocholithiasis, cholangitis, acute pancreatitis, intestinal obstruction, diverticulitis, peritonitis, perforation, gastritis, ulcer, constipation
- Urogenital: renal colic, testicular torsion, acute bladder retention, urinary tract infection (UTI), acute pelvic inflammatory disease (PID), ectopic pregnancy, ovarian torsion
- Vascular: abdominal aortic aneurysm (AAA), dissection, mesenteric ischaemia, ischaemic colitis

Extra-abdominal

- Adrenal insufficiency
- Abdominal wall: herpes zoster, muscle haematoma, hernia, anterior cutaneous nerve entrapment syndrome (ACNES)
- Cardiopulmonary: acute coronary syndrome (ACS), pneumonia, pulmonary embolism
- Metabolic: diabetic ketoacidosis (DKA), alcoholic ketoacidosis

External notification*

- *High urgency* → care for patient in trauma room, inform the emergency team and triage nurse, register with secretary
- *Low urgency* → care for patient in standard room, register with secretary

* Estimate based on information received about transfer

Internal notification*

- *High urgency* → telephonic instructions + immediate assessment
- *Low urgency* → telephonic instructions + assess in the near future AB

* Estimate based on information received about handover

Instructions regarding initial care in emergency department (ED)

- Continuous monitoring of vital signs
- Cannula + lab tests as indicated: blood count, diff, CRP, electrolytes, renal function, lactate, glucose, troponine, CK, liver enzymes, amylase or lipase, arterial blood gas (ABG), cross-match serum, blood cultures
- Examination of the abdomen
- 12-lead ECG
- Urine sediment
- For women of child-bearing age: pregnancy test

Instructions regarding initial care on nursing ward

- Second nurse in the room
- Create calm/space to work
- COW in the room, patient details on stand-by
- Vital signs every 15-30 min
- Examination of the abdomen
- Contact on-call doctor immediately if patient deteriorates

Continue initial care on the nursing ward, doctor on scene

- Cannula + lab tests as indicated: blood count, diff, CRP, electrolytes, renal function, lactate, glucose, troponine, CK, liver enzymes, amylase or lipase, ABG, cross-match serum, blood cultures
- 12-lead ECG
- Urine sediment
- For women of child-bearing age: pregnancy test

Recommendations following assessment

- Use ABCDE approach
- Consider chest X-ray, urgent ultrasound (FAST) by ED doctor (assess for free fluid, aneurysm), abdominal ultrasound, abdominal CT
- Consult surgeon/gynaecologist/gastro-enterologist sooner rather than later
- If the patient is on a nursing ward, request early consultation by ERT
- Specific treatment instructions are provided in the section *Conditions*

Diagram 8 // Management of a patient with altered or decreased consciousness

The management of a patient with altered* or a decreased consciousness

* Altered consciousness refers to a change in consciousness. A change in consciousness does not necessarily imply a reduced level of consciousness!

↓

Consider at least the following

- Cardiovascular: shock, circulatory arrest
- Delirium
- Intoxications: medication (benzodiazepines, opiates, antidepressants), drugs (downers: GHB, alcohol, opiates, heroin; trippers: LSD, magic mushrooms; uppers: XTC, cocaine)
- Metabolic: hypoglycaemia, electrolyte imbalances, hepatic coma, hypothermia/hyperthermia, thyroid disorders
- Neurological: intracranial haemorrhage (SAB, SDH, EDH), ischaemic/haemorrhagic stroke, meningitis, encephalitis, seizures, space-occupying lesion (SOL)
- Psychiatric: psychosis, schizophrenia, personality disorders
- Respiratory: respiratory insufficiency (hypoxia, hypercapnia)
- Sepsis

External notification

High urgency → care for patient in trauma room, inform emergency team and triage nurse, register with secretary

Internal notification

High urgency → telephonic instructions + immediate assessment

Instructions regarding initial care in ED

- Explicit focus on the airway
- Direct bedside glucose, treat hypoglycaemia
- Continuous monitoring of vital signs
- ABG
- Cannula + lab tests as indicated: blood count, diff, CRP, lactate, glucose, electrolytes, liver enzymes, ammonia, tox screen
- In case of potential infection: start AB after collecting blood/ urine cultures

Recommendations following assessment

- Use ABCDE approach
- If necessary, implement measures to secure the airway
- Consider brain CT
- Consider lumbar puncture (after ruling out risk of herniation by means of brain CT)
- For severe hypoglycaemia: administer 10g glucose as a slow bolus IV (10g = 100 mL gluc 10% = 20 mL gluc 50%: expected increase of 2 mmol/L per 10g) and check glucose <10 min, repeat if necessary
- Complete the Delirium Observation Screening (DOS)
- If the patient is on a nursing ward, request early consultation by ERT
- Specific treatment instructions are provided in the section *Conditions*

Instructions regarding initial care on nursing ward

- Second nurse in the room
- Create calm/space to work
- COW in the room, patient details on stand-by
- Explicit focus on the airway
- Direct bedside glucose, treat hypoglycaemia
- Vital signs every 5 min
- Insert + flush cannula
- Have materials for ABG/lab tests present
- Contact on-call doctor immediately if patient deteriorates

Continue initial care on the nursing ward, doctor on scene

- ABG by doctor
- Lab tests as indicated: blood count, diff, CRP, lactate, glucose, electrolytes, liver enzymes, ammonia, tox screen

Diagram 9 // Management of a patient with an arrhythmia

The management of a patient with arrhythmia

Actively search for presence of any unfavourable signs (high urgency)

- HF
- Myocardial ischaemia
- Shock (systolic BP <90 mmHg)
- Syncope

External notification*

- *High urgency* → care for patient in trauma room, inform emergency team and triage nurse, register with secretary
- *Low urgency* → care for patient in standard room, register with secretary

* Estimate based on information received about transfer

Instructions regarding initial care in ED

- Continuous monitoring of vital signs
- 12-lead ECG + rhythm strip
- Cannula + lab tests as indicated: blood count, CRP, electrolytes, renal function, TSH. Consider tox screen.
- Ensure a defibrillator within reach in case of (stable) VT

Internal notification*

- *High urgency* → telephonic instructions + immediate assessment
- *Low urgency* → telephonic instructions + assess in the near future

* Estimate based on information received about transfer

Instructions regarding initial care on nursing ward

- Second nurse in the room
- Create calm/space to work
- COW in the room, patient details on stand-by
- Monitor vital signs at an appropriate frequency
- 12-lead ECG + rhythm strip
- Cannula + lab tests as indicated: blood count, CRP, electrolytes, renal function, TSH. Consider tox screen.
- Contact on-call doctor immediately if patient deteriorates

Recommendations following assessment

- Use ABCDE approach → if the patient exhibits any unfavourable signs, call for assistance immediately (ED doctor/cardiologist/ICU specialist)
- The frequency at which vital signs such as blood pressure should be determined depends on the clinical presentation and whether or not the patient is stable
- Consult with the cardiologist, treat according to the algorithm bradycardia/tachycardia (Diagram 10 and 24)
- If the patient is on a nursing ward, request early consultation by ERT
- Specific treatment instructions are provided in the section *Conditions*

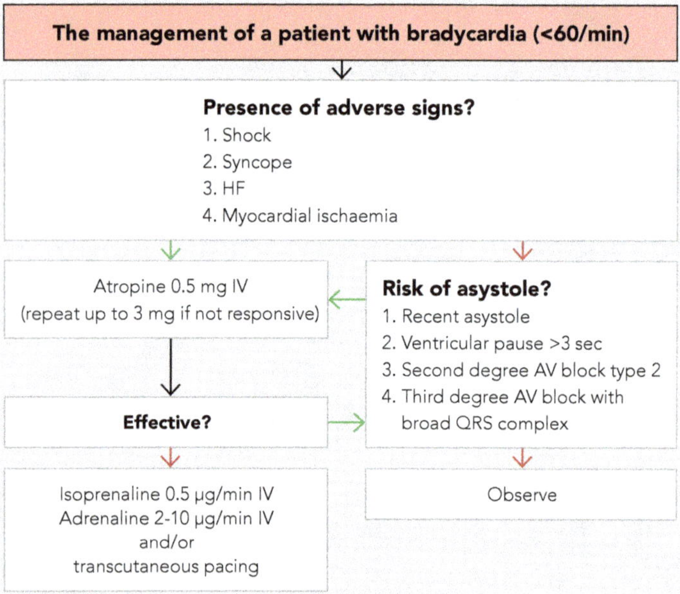

Diagram 10 // Management of a patient with bradycardia

TIMING FOR CT SCAN	CRITERIA BRAIN CT
<1h	• GCS ≤12 on initial assessment • GCS <15 2h after injury • Focal neurological deficits • >1 episode of vomiting • Post-traumatic seizure • Suspected open or depressed skull fracture • Sign of basal skull fracture (e.g. battle sign, CSF leakage from ear/nose, bilateral periorbital haematoma, haemotympanum)
<8h*	Loss of consciousness or amnesia and one of the following: • Age ≥65 • Coagulopathy/anticoagulant**/antiplatelet therapy (excluding acetylsalicylic acid monotherapy) • Dangerous mechanism of injury • >30 min retrograde amnesia

Table 67 // Indications brain CT after TBI in patients ≥16y

Please note: brain CT is recommended if any one of the criteria is met

* Or <1h in case of delayed presentation (>8h after injury)

** Anticoagulant treatment includes VKAs, DOACs or (low-molecular-weight) heparins

The management of a patient with discoloration of extremities

↓

Location

Unilateral discoloration
- Cellulitis/erysipelas
- Critical limb ischaemia secondary to peripheral vascular disease (acute arterial occlusion due to arterial embolism, atherosclerosis, Buerger disease) → URGENT!
- Venous stasis/occlusion (e.g. DVT)

Bilateral discoloration
- Cardiac output ↓ due to HF or shock → URGENT!
- Central cyanosis
- Hyperviscosity (i.e. due to multiple myeloma, polycythaemia, macroglobulinemia)
- Local vasoconstriction due to cold exposure (hypothermia)
- Vasomotor instability

↓

Assessment advice:
1. Assess patient according to ABCDE approach
2. Check arterial pulsations (compared with Doppler test)
3. Additional diagnostics:
   - Doppler test: demonstrate arterial blood flow in distal extremities
   - Consider ECG, chest X-ray, chest CT: to exclude cardiopulmonary cause
   - Consider ankle-brachial index (ABI) and consider CTA/duplex ultrasound: detect arterial stenosis or DVT
   - Consider D-dimer: to exclude the likelihood of venous thrombus
   - CRP to exclude an infectious cause for discoloration

Diagram 11 // Management of a patient with discoloration of extremities

In case of discoloration of distal extremities, lips, nose, earlobes, and oral cavity, consider central cyanosis.

Diagram 12 // Management of a patient with chest pain

The management of a patient with chest pain

Consider at least the following
- Cardiovascular: acute coronary syndrome, tamponade, pericarditis, aortic dissection
- Pulmonary: pneumonia, pulmonary embolism, pneumothorax, pleuritis
- Chest wall: costochondral/myofascial, herpes zoster
- Gastrointestinal/abdominal: stomach problems, ventricular/duodenal ulcer, cholecystitis, cholelithiasis, pancreatitis, reflux oesophagitis, oesophageal rupture

External notification*
- *High urgency* → care for patient in trauma room, inform emergency team and triage nurse, register with secretary
- *Low urgency* → care for patient in standard room, register with secretary

* Estimate based on information received about transfer

Internal notification*
- *High urgency* → telephonic instructions + immediate assessment
- *Low urgency* → telephonic instructions + assess in the near future

* Estimate based on information received about transfer

Instructions regarding initial care in ED
- Continuous monitoring of vital signs
- Immediate 12-lead ECG
- Cannula + lab tests: blood count, electrolytes, renal function, transaminases, amylase or lipase, CK, CK-MB, LDH, CRP, troponine, coagulation and possibly D-dimer
- Chest X-ray

Instructions regarding initial care on nursing ward
- Second nurse in the room
- Create calm/space to work
- COW in the room, patient details on stand-by
- Immediate 12-lead ECG
- Vital signs every 10 min

- Cannula + lab tests: blood count, electrolytes, renal function, transaminases, amylase or lipase, CK, CK-MB, LDH, CRP, troponine, coagulation and possibly D-dimer
- Contact on-call doctor immediately if patient deteriorates

Continue initial care on the nursing ward, doctor on scene

- Chest X-ray (bedside if necessary)

Recommendations following assessment

- Use ABCDE approach
- Suspected ACS: caution is advised when administering O2 (damage caused by hyperoxia, target saturation 94-98%, or 88-92% for COPD with unknown baseline saturation) and large volumes of IV fluids (risk of HF); in the case of cardiogenic shock, consider ionotropics → consult cardiologist/ICU specialist
- Suspected (tension) pneumothorax: indication for decompression via needle thoracocentesis → call for help immediately (ED doctor/ERT)
- Check blood pressure and peripheral pulsations on both sides, to detect possible dissection of thoracic aorta
- Consider urgent ultrasound: ventricular function, tamponade, right-sided HF, pneumothorax, intimal flap with aortic dissection
- Compare the current ECG to an old ECG: are these new or pre-existing abnormalities?
- Repeat ECG after 30 min: are there any visible changes compared to original ECG (immediate dynamics)?
- CT pulmonary angiogram (CTPA), if a pulmonary embolism is suspected
- Specific treatment instructions are provided in the section *Conditions*

The management of a patient with deterioration after surgery

1. Assess patient according to ABCDE approach
2. Assess surgical site (e.g. discoloration, bleeding, infection)
3. Assess input and output values:
   - IV fluid intake and urine output
   - Surgical drain output volume and appearance (if applicable)
   - Stool output (e.g. none, mucus, melaena)
4. Check previous (postoperative) lab results, cultures, medication, imaging or operation reports

Potential complications (e.g.)

- Drug-induced (e.g. opioids, AKI)
- Fluid imbalance
- Haemorrhage or thrombosis
- Infection or sepsis
- Surgery specific complications (e.g. anastomotic leak, bowel obstruction, compartment syndrome)

Request additional diagnostics

Indicated laboratory exams and/or imaging matching your differential diagnosis (e.g. Hb, blood group, CRP, lactate, renal function, POCUS, chest X-ray, abdominal CT)

Infection

Sepsis (qSOFA ≥2/3 criteria):

- Systolic blood pressure <100 mmHg
- Respiratory rate >20/min
- GCS <15

Postoperative haemorrhage / thrombosis

Postoperative haemorrhage:

- Local haemorrhage
- Haemorrhagic stroke

Diagram 13 // Management of a patient with deterioration after surgery

Postoperative fever (T>38.5°C) → evaluate possible cause (5W):

- Wind: pneumonia
- Water: urinary tract infection
- Walking: DVT, pulmonary embolism
- Wound: infection, resorption response of large hematomas
- Wonder drugs: medication

↓

- 2 sets of blood cultures, consider additional cultures like sputum and wound culture
- Treatment of underlying cause (e.g. targeted AB: broad spectrum or based on cultures)
- Supportive care (e.g. IV fluids)

Thrombotic complications:

- DVT
- Ischaemic stroke
- Portal vein thrombosis
- Pulmonary embolism

↓

Haemorrhage

- Adjustment of pharmacological treatment (e.g. stop anticoagulants, start 4-factor prothrombin complex concentrate)
- Treatment of bleeding focus (surgery or IV embolisation)

Thrombosis

- Start therapeutic dose of anticoagulants
- Possible thrombosuction or IVT (e.g. intracranial thrombus or central pulmonary embolism)

↓

Fluid imbalance

- AKI
- Diarrhoea
- Excessive administration of IV fluid
- Excessive surgical drain output
- Excessive vomiting
- Haemorrhage
- HF
- Urinary retention

↓

Fluid resuscitation

- V fluids
- Monitor input and output

! Fluid overload (esp. in patients with heart- or kidney failure)

The management of a patient after a fall out of bed

↓

1. Assess ABCDE (extra attention for C-spine) → if unstable first stabilise the patient
2. Was there loss of consciousness prior to the fall? If yes, perform analysis for syncope (e.g. ECG)
3. Has the patient fallen on his head? If yes, consider brain CT (see Table 67)
4. Is there suspicion for a fracture? If yes, consider radiography

↓

Consider the following causes (the following conditions can present as a fall):

↓

Transient loss of consciousness/altered consciousness

- Delirium
- Hypovolemia
- Infection/sepsis
- Ischaemic/haemorrhagic stroke
- Medication (e.g. use of opiates, antihypertensives, benzodiazepines)
- Metabolic derangements
- Orthostatic hypotension
- Seizure
- Vasovagal response

No loss of consciousness

- ACS
- Arrhythmia
- Ischaemic stroke/transient ischaemic attack (TIA)
- Pulmonary embolism

Other causes

- Different environment
- Not wearing shoes/wearing slippery shoes or socks

Diagram 14 // Management of a patient after a fall out of bed

Physical examination
- Neurological assessment
- Inspection for wounds
- Assessment of extremities and spine (e.g. fracture)

Consider additional diagnostics
- ECG for syncope
- Labs (e.g. D-dimer for thromboembolism)
- X-ray to exclude a fracture
- Brain CT to exclude intracranial haemorrhage

Assess fall risk *(the following factors increase fall risk)***:**
- Age >80
- Medication:
  - Polypharmacy → minimise the number of different medications used if possible
  - Medication that increases fall risk (e.g. benzodiazepines, antidepressants, alpha- and beta blockers, antihypertensives, alpha blocking agents, opiates)
- Underlying medical conditions (e.g. orthostatic hypotension, gait difficulties, arthritis)

In increased risk: discuss fall prevention strategies and provide general education.
In case of (increased risk of) delirium: take delirium prevention and management precautions.

Diagram 15 // Management of a patient with dyspnoea

The management of a patient with dyspnoea

↓

Consider at least the following

- Pulmonary: upper airway cause (e.g. infection, anaphylaxis), (tension) pneumothorax, pulmonary embolism, pneumonia, asthma/COPD flare-up, pleural effusion
- Respiratory insufficiency resulting from pneumothorax, pneumonia, atelectasis, asthma/COPD flare-up, multiple rib fractures, haemothorax, diaphragmatic paralysis (e.g. Guillain-Barré Syndrome)
- Cardiac: ischaemia/infarction, arrhythmia, decompensated HF (DHF), valve disease, myocarditis
- Metabolic: metabolic acidosis, hyperthyroidism, anaemia, sepsis
- Psychological: anxiety/panic attack

↓

External notification*

- *High urgency* → care for patient in trauma room, inform emergency team and triage nurse, register with secretary
- *Low urgency* → care for patient in standard room, register with secretary

* Estimate based on information received about transfer

↓

Instructions regarding initial care in ED

- Continuous monitoring of vital signs
- Start O_2 based on saturation
- ABG
- Chest X-ray

↓

Internal notification*

- *High urgency* → telephonic instructions + immediate assessment
- *Low urgency* → telephonic instructions + assess in the near future

* Estimate based on information received about transfer

↓

Instructions regarding initial care on nursing ward

- Second nurse in the room
- Create calm/space to work
- COW in the room, patient details on stand-by
- Vital signs every 10 min
- Start O_2 based on saturation

- Consider ultrasound examination of the chest according to BLUE protocol (Bedside Lung Ultrasound in Emergency, applied for acute respiratory failure)
- Cannula + lab tests as indicated: blood count, renal function, lactate, glucose, D-dimer, CRP, troponine, CK, NT-pro-BNP
- 12-lead ECG

Recommendations following assessment

- Use ABCDE approach
- Signs of respiratory insufficiency/need for respiratory support → call for help immediately (ED doctor/ERT)
- Suspected (tension) pneumothorax: indication for decompression via needle thoracocentesis → call for help immediately (ED doctor/ERT)
- Bronchospasms: nebuliser treatment with salbutamol/ipratropium bromide, consider corticosteroids and AB → consult Respiratory Medicine specialist sooner rather than later
- Acute HF: furosemide IV for afterload reduction, consider adding nitroglycerin if blood pressure permits. In the case of respiratory insufficiency or inadequate response to previous interventions, you can start NIV. Contact the cardiologist or the ERT sooner rather than later.
- Specific treatment instructions are provided in the section *Conditions*

- 12-lead ECG
- Have materials for AEG/lab tests present
- Contact on-call doctor immediately if patient deteriorates

Continue initial care on the nursing ward, doctor on scene

- ABG by doctor
- Cannula + lab tests as indicated: blood count, renal function, lactate, glucose, D-dimer, CRP, troponine, CK, NT-pro-BNP
- Chest X-ray (bedside if necessary, depending on options to move the patient)

In practice, it is becoming increasingly common to collect a venous gas sample instead of an arterial gas sample. A conversion table provides reliable estimates of, among others, the arterial pCO_2, after which the gas value can be interpreted as usual in ASA 1 patients.

Diagram 16 // Management of a patient with headache

The management of a patient with headache

Consider at least the following

- Primary types of headache: migraine, tension headache, cluster headache
- Secondary types of headache: SAB, SDH, EDH, stroke, hypertensive crisis, meningitis, encephalitis, trigeminal neuralgia, giant cell arthritis, acute glaucoma, increased intracranial pressure, viral infection, sinusitis, dehydration, sleep deprivation, medication induced

External notification*

- *High urgency* → care for patient in trauma room, inform emergency team and triage nurse, register with secretary
- *Low urgency* → care for patient in standard room, register with secretary

* Estimate based on information received about transfer

Internal notification*

- *High urgency* → telephonic instructions + immediate assessment
- *Low urgency* → telephonic instructions + assess in the near future

* Estimate based on information received about transfer

Instructions regarding initial care in ED

- Continuous monitoring of vital signs
- Cannula + lab tests as indicated: blood count, CRP, renal function, coagulation and BSE
- Provide pain medication if necessary
- In case of potential meningitis: start AB

Instructions regarding initial care on nursing ward

- Second nurse in the room
- Create calm/space to work
- COW in the room, patient details on stand-by
- Vital signs every 10-30 min
- Contact on-call doctor immediately if patient deteriorates

Continue initial care on the nursing ward, doctor on scene

- Cannula + lab tests as indicated: blood count, CRP, renal function, coagulation

Recommendations following assessment

- Use ABCDE approach
- Perform a complete neurological examination during the secondary survey
- Consider brain CT
- Consider lumbar puncture (after ruling out risk of herniation by means of brain CT)
- Suspected stroke: consult a neurologist immediately, to consider potential IAT or IVT
- Suspected SAH: consult a neurologist and consider a CTA of the brain to assess vascular malformations
- Suspected hypertensive crisis: consult ophthalmologist to assess for retinopathy, smear for fragmentocytes (for DDx HUS/TTP), ECG, troponine, CK, urine for protein. Treat as an "emergency" if there are any signs of organ damage → aim for blood pressure reduction (max 25%) within several minutes to hours using IV medication on a monitored ward
- Consult a neurologist/neurosurgeon sooner rather than later
- Specific treatment instructions are provided in the section *Conditions*

Diagram 17 // Management of a patient with hyperthermia

The management of a patient with hyperthermia*

*An increase in the temperature set point by endogenous or exogenous mediators is referred to as a fever

↓

Consider at least the following

- Acute bacterial/viral/fungal infection
- Anticholinergic syndrome
- Drug fever
- Malignancy
- Post-operative
- Serotonergic syndrome/malignant neuroleptic syndrome
- Thrombo-embolism
- Thyrotoxic crisis (thyroid storm)
- Transfusion reaction

↓

External notification*

- *High urgency* → care for patient in trauma room, inform emergency team and triage nurse, register with secretary
- *Low urgency* → care for patient in standard room, register with secretary

* Estimate based on information received about transfer

Internal notification*

- *High urgency* → telephonic instructions + immediate assessment
- *Low urgency* → telephonic instructions + assess in the near future

* Estimate based on information received about transfer

Instructions regarding initial care in ED

- Continuous monitoring of vital signs
- Cannula + lab tests as indicated: blood count, diff, CRP, lactate, glucose, blood cultures
- Urine sediment and cultures
- Chest X-ray or POCUS

Instructions regarding initial care on nursing ward

- Second nurse in the room
- Create calm/space to work
- COW in the room, patient details on stand-by
- Vital signs every 10-30 min
- Cannula + lab tests as indicated: blood count, diff, CRP, lactate, glucose, blood cultures
- Urine sediment and cultures
- Contact on-call doctor immediately if patient deteriorates

Continue initial care on the nursing ward, doctor on scene

- Chest X-ray (bedside if necessary)

Recommendations following assessment

- Use ABCDE approach
- Consider (timely) administration of AB
- If the patient has clinical signs of shock and does not respond to IV fluids, consider corticosteroids
- If the patient is on a nursing ward, request early consultation by ERT
- Specific treatment instructions are provided in the section *Conditions*

Diagram 18 // Management of a patient with neurological deficits

The management of a patient with neurological deficits

↓

Consider at least the following

- Traumatic: subdural/epidural haematoma
- Vascular: TIA/ischaemic stroke, SAH, dissection of aorta/carotid artery/vertebral artery, hypertensive encephalopathy, vasculitis, haemorrhagic stroke
- Neoplastic: SOL
- Other: migraine
- Idiopathic: peripheral facial paralysis
- Infectious: meningitis, encephalitis, intracranial abscess
- Metabolic: hyperglycaemia/hypoglycaemia, hypernatraemia/hyponatraemia, hepatic encephalopathy

↓

External notification

High urgency → care for patient in trauma room, inform emergency team and triage nurse, register with secretary

Internal notification

High urgency → telephonic instructions + immediate assessment

Instructions regarding initial care in ED

- Continuous monitoring of vital signs
- Cannula + lab tests as indicated: blood count, coagulation, CRP, electrolytes, renal function, liver enzymes, lactate, glucose

Instructions regarding initial care on nursing ward

- Second nurse in the room
- Create calm/space to work
- COW in the room, patient details on stand-by
- Vital signs every 10 min
- Cannula + lab tests as indicated: blood count, CRP, coagulation, electrolytes, renal function, liver enzymes, lactate, glucose
- Contact on-call doctor immediately if patient deteriorates

Recommendations following assessment

- Use ABCDE approach
- Respond quickly: time is brain!
- Correct hypoglycaemia: glucose 20 mL 50%, check glucose <10 min, repeat if necessary. N.B.: In the case of a suspected thiamine deficiency, first administer 250-500mg thiamine after drawing blood for vitamin B1 tests IV or IM before administering glucose (dose depends on estimate of severity).
- Consult a neurologist immediately → indication for IAT or IVT?
- If the patient is on a nursing ward, request early consultation by ERT or the neurologist
- Specific treatment instructions are provided in the section *Conditions*

Diagram 19 // Management of a patient with an obstructed airway

The management of a patient with an obstructed airway

↓

Consider at least the following

- Airway obstruction caused by foreign body, blood/vomit, soft tissue swelling, trauma
- Decreased consciousness caused by trauma, intoxication, ischaemic/haemorrhagic stroke, hypercapnia, metabolic cause (hypoglycaemia, hepatic encephalopathy)

External notification

High urgency → care for patient in trauma room, inform emergency team and triage nurse, register with secretary

Instructions regarding initial care in ED

- Provide care jointly with an experienced emergency team preferably incl. an anaesthesiologist. Whilst waiting for the patient, conduct a short briefing with the team → start with clear task allocation. If a potentially "difficult" airway is suspected, report this immediately.
- Airway management materials (suction system + Yankauer, Guedell, (video) laryngoscope, Ambu bag) close at hand
- Continuous monitoring of vital signs
- Chest X-ray, if indicated
- Insert + flush cannula

Internal notification

High urgency → telephonic instructions + immediate assessment, (ask someone to) inform supervisor without delay

Instructions regarding initial care on nursing ward

- Real suspicion of airway obstruction → IMMEDIATELY call for the resuscitation team, have someone wait for the team at the entrance to the ward
- If a potentially "difficult" airway is suspected, report this immediately to whoever you have called in to help
- Second nurse in the room
- Continuous registration of saturation and rhythm if possible, check vital signs at least every minute
- Airway management materials (suction system + Yankauer, Guedell, Ambu bag) close at hand

- Lab tests, if indicated: ABG, glucose, blood count, CRP, tox screen
- Suspected circulatory arrest secondary to airway problem
  → IMMEDIATELY start BLS and call for the ER

- Insert + flush cannula
- Create calm/space to work, remove headboard from bed, move bed away from the wall
- COW in the room, patient details on stand-by
- If you suspect a circulatory arrest and are still waiting for the doctor → IMMEDIATELY start BLS + call for the ERT

Recommendations following assessment

- Use ABCDE approach
- Suspected foreign body and responsive patient
  → Coughing: stimulate coughing
  → Not coughing (effectively): apply five firm slaps with a flat hand between the shoulder blades, alternating with five abdominal thrusts (Heimlich)
- Other suspected causes and/or non-responsive patient
  → Jaw-thrust by doctor, suction of semi-solid debris by nurse if necessary
  → Airway (partially) free after manual manoeuvre (+ suction): support breathing by means of two-person technique (beware of hyperinflation). Administer additional O_2, consider using Guedell.
- Formally hand over to the resuscitation team when they arrive and remain in the room for further assistance
- Specific treatment instructions are provided in the section *Conditions*

Diagram 20 // Management of a patient with seizures

The management of a patient with seizures

Consider at least the following
- Primary epilepsy
- Secondary epilepsy: traumatic brain injury, intracranial bleeding, infection (meningitis, encephalitis, abscess), metabolic abnormalities (hypoglycaemia/hyperglycaemia, hyponatraemia/hypernatraemia, uraemia, hepatic encephalopathy), intoxications (cocaine, antidepressants, alcohol withdrawal), hypertensive encephalopathy, malignant neuroleptic syndrome

External notification

High urgency → care for patient in trauma room, inform emergency team and triage nurse, register with secretary

Instructions regarding initial care in ED
- Continuous monitoring of vital signs
- Cannula + lab tests as indicated: blood count, liver enzymes, CRP, NA, K, Ca, Mg, phosphate, glucose, renal function, CK, consider checking concentrations of anti-epileptics and/or tox screen

Internal notification

High urgency → telephonic instructions + immediate assessment

Instructions regarding initial care on nursing ward
- Second nurse in the room
- Create calm/space to work
- COW in the room, patient details on stand-by
- Vital signs every 10 min
- Have materials for ABG/lab tests present
- Contact on-call doctor immediately if patient deteriorates

Continue initial care on the nursing ward, doctor on scene

- Cannula + lab tests as indicated: blood count, GGT, ALAT, CRP, electrolytes, Ca, Mg, phosphate, glucose, renal function, CK, consider checking concentrations of anti-epileptics and/or tox screen

↓

Recommendations following assessment

- Use ABCDE approach
- For treatment recommendation, see diagram 21 on next page
- For status epilepticus: consider intubation
- Watch out for aspiration → consider a chest X-ray
- Correct hypoglycaemia: glucose 20 mL 50%, check glucose <10 min, repeat if necessary.
  N.B.: In the case of a suspected thiamine deficiency, first administer 250-500 mg thiamine IV or IM before administering glucose (dose depends on estimate of severity).
- Consult a neurologist/ERT sooner rather than later
- Specific treatment instructions are provided in the section *Conditions*

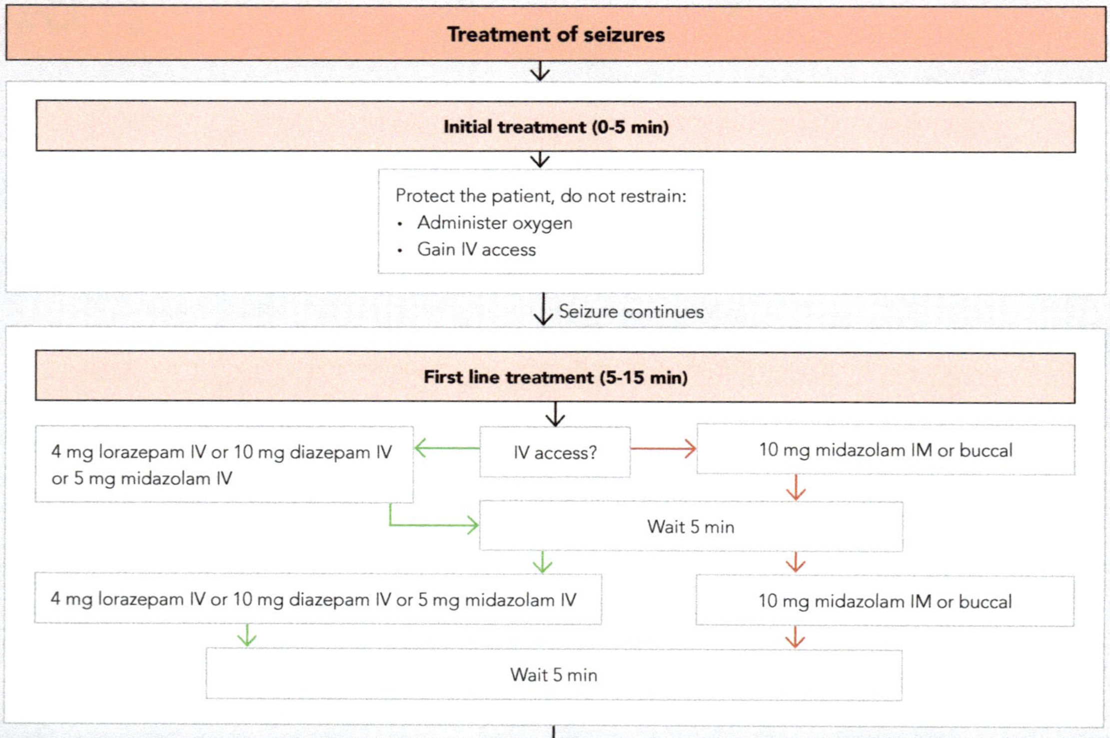

Diagram 21 // Treatment of seizures

Seizure continues

Second line treatment (15+ min)

Get IV or IO access!

IV levetiracetam 60 mg/kg

- Max. 4500 mg (in sodium chloride 0.9% over 10 min)
- Levetiracetam is preferred in polypharmacy since it has the fewest drug interactions

IV phenytoin 20 mg/kg

- Max. 2g (rate 50 mg/min, 25 mg/min for elderly or patients with cardiac history, give undiluted)
- When administering phenytoin, cardiac monitoring has to be available

IV valproate 40 mg/kg

- Max. 3000 mg (in 100 ml NaCl 0.9% over 5 min)
- Valproate is preferred for generalised epilepsy. Be careful administering to potentially childbearing patients (teratogenic).

If the seizure continues after administrating one of three above, consider giving a different IV anti-epileptic drug from the list above OR phenobarbital (15 mg/kg as a single dose, max. rate 100 mg/min)

If you are approaching 30 min of seizures, contact your supervisor and critical care

When seizure stops

- Use ABCDE approach
- Consider transfer to critical care
- Start supportive medical care and look for underlying causes of seizure

Diagram 22 // Management of a patient with shock symptoms

The management of a patient exhibiting shock symptoms

Consider at least the following
- Cardiogenic shock: infarction, arrhythmia, HF
- Distributive shock: sepsis, anaphylaxis, adrenal insufficiency, neurogenic
- Hypovolaemic shock: severe dehydration, bleeding
- Obstructive shock: tamponade, tension pneumothorax, massive pulmonary embolism

External notification*
- *High urgency* → care for patient in trauma room, inform emergency team and triage nurse, register with secretary
- *Low urgency* → care for patient in standard room, register with secretary

* Estimate based on information received about transfer

Internal notification*
- *High urgency* → telephonic instructions + immediate assessment
- *Low urgency* → telephonic instructions + assess in the near future

* Estimate based on information received about transfer

Instructions regarding initial care in ED
- Continuous monitoring of vital signs
- Two well-functioning IV's
- Lab tests as indicated: blood count, blood group, cross-match serum, electrolytes, renal function, lactate, D-dimer, CRP, troponine, CK, coagulation tests
- Two sets of blood cultures, urine and sputum culture
- 12-lead ECG
- Chest X-ray, POCUS RUSH protocol

Instructions regarding initial care on nursing ward
- Second nurse in the room
- Create calm/space to work
- COW in the room, patient details on stand-by
- Vital signs every 5-10 min
- Two well-functioning IV's
- Lab tests as indicated: blood count, blood group, cross-match serum, electrolytes, renal function, lactate, D-dimer, CRP, troponine, CK

- Two sets of blood cultures, urine and sputum culture
- 12-lead ECG
- Contact on-call doctor immediately if patient deteriorates

Continue initial care on the nursing ward, doctor on scene

- Chest X-ray (bedside if necessary)

Recommendations following assessment

- Use ABCDE approach
- Suspected sepsis: start broad-spectrum AB as soon as possible after collecting cultures
- Fluid challenge NaCl 0.9% or Ringer's lactate (except for cardiogenic shock → consult with ICU about starting ionotropics). Consider the massive blood loss protocol for shock caused by bleeding.
- Consider an urgent ultrasound according to the RUSH protocol (Rapid Ultrasound in Shock)
- Suspected adrenal insufficiency: 100 mg hydrocortisone IV
- Suspected (tension) pneumothorax: indication for decompression via needle thoracocentesis → call for help immediately (ED doctor/ERT)
- Suspected pericardial tamponade: indication for pericardiocentesis → call for help immediately (ED doctor/ERT/cardiologist)
- Suspected anaphylaxis: 0.5 mg adrenaline IM
- Suspected massive pulmonary embolism: IVT, admission to monitored ward. Consult ICU specialist.
- Underlying arrhythmia: manage according to resuscitation algorithm
- If indicated, indwelling catheter + urine flow meter, start monitoring fluid balance
- If the patient is on a nursing ward, request early consultation by ERT
- Specific treatment instructions are provided in the section *Conditions*

The management of a patient with syncope

Consider at least the following
- Cardiovascular: arrhythmias, HF, pulmonary embolism, aortic valve stenosis
- Medication: antihypertensives
- Orthostatic hypotension: hypovolaemia, age, comorbidities, medication
- Reflex-mediated: vasovagal, situational (e.g. after micturition)

External notification
Low urgency → care for patient in standard room, register with secretary

Instructions regarding initial care in ED
- Continuous monitoring of vital signs (rhythm monitoring)
- Cannula + lab tests only if indicated
- 12-lead ECG, repeat if symptoms recur

Internal notification
Low urgency → telephonic instructions + assess in the near future

Instructions regarding initial care on nursing ward
- Second nurse in the room
- Create calm/space to work
- COW in the room, patient details on stand-by
- Vital signs every 10 min
- 12-lead ECG, repeat if symptoms recur
- Consider consulting ERT/transfer to monitored ward for rhythm observation
- Contact on-call doctor immediately if patient deteriorates

Continue initial care on the nursing ward, doctor on scene
- Cannula + lab tests only if indicated

Recommendations following assessment
- Use ABCDE approach
- Measure orthostasis (lying down and then after standing for 3 min). Orthostasis is defined as a drop in BP >20 mmHg systolic and/or 10 mg diastolic <3 min after standing. Enquire about co-existing and prodromal symptoms.
- Try to estimate the patient's fluid intake status
- Specific treatment instructions are provided in the section *Conditions*

Diagram 23 // Management of a patient with syncope

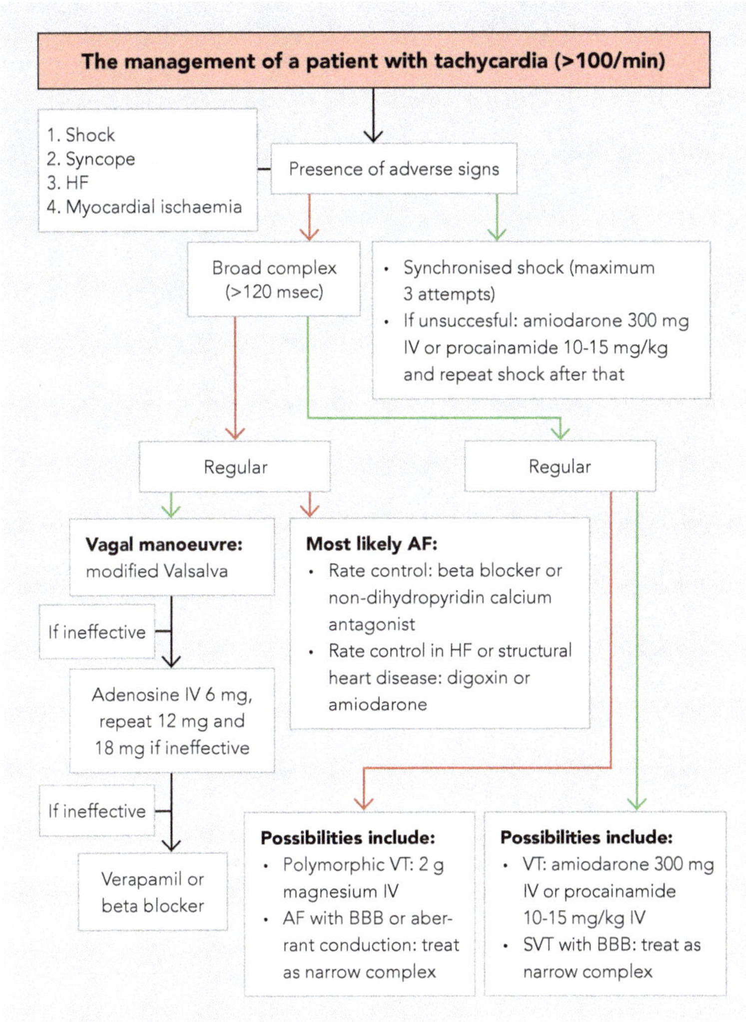

Diagram 24 // Management of a patient with tachycardia

Please ask the time of the patient's last meal. If the patient has not fasted, the anaesthesiologist will need to perform intubation prior to cardioversion to prevent aspiration.

Diagram 25 // Management of a patient with wounds

The management of a patient with wounds

Consider the following
- What's the extent of injury?
- What's the degree of contamination?
- Is there injury to adjacent neurovascular structures and bones?

Acute wound: identifiable mechanism of injury (e.g. trauma, surgical) leading to skin disruption/damage (watch for dehiscence i.e. Platzbauch in postoperative patients)

Chronic wound: arrested during normal stages of healing (>3 mo of non-progression, e.g., ulcer)

Consider the following causes:
- Arterial (i.e. arterial ulcer) → consider ABI
- Venous (i.e. venous ulcer)
- Systemic (e.g. diabetic ulcer)
- Infection (e.g. cellulitis, erysipelas) → collect culture
- Pressure wound
- Other (e.g. radiation, oncological, pharmacological, smoking)

Treatment (TIME clinical decision tool)**:**
1. Ensure tissue viability
   - Black wound (necrosis) → necrotomy
2. Manage infection/inflammation
   - Yellow wound (infection) → consider AB
3. Manage moisture imbalance
   - Red wound (granulation) → protect
4. Optimise edges of wound

Open: skin breakage, exposure to outside environment

Consider the cause (e.g. laceration, stabwound, abrasion, gunshot)

Assess underlying tissue/neurovascular structures (e.g. risk of tendon injury, pneumothorax)

Treatment:
- Irrigation and debridement
- Primary closure for clean, uninfected wound with approximable edges
- Secondary/tertiary closure for all other wounds
- Consider AB in high risk of infection (e.g. injury to tendons, visual bone tissue)

Closed: no skin breakage

Consider the cause (e.g. haematoma, contusion, blunt trauma)

Treatment:
- Screen for complications (e.g. DVT)
- Minimise further inflammation: POLICE

TIME wound management
- **T**issue: viable or deficient
- **I**nfection or inflammation
- **M**oisture: imbalance
- **E**dge: non-advancing or undermined

POLICE:
- **P**rotection
- **O**ptimal **L**oading
- **I**ce
- **C**ompression
- **E**levation

Conditions

Cardiology and vascular medicine

Acute coronary syndrome

	UNSTABLE ANGINA PECTORIS	NON-ST ELEVATION MYOCARDIAL INFARCTION (NSTEMI)	ST ELEVATION MYOCARDIAL INFARCTION (STEMI)
D	Characterised by an increase in ischaemic symptoms manifesting as anginal symptoms at rest, new anginal symptoms, and increasing anginal symptoms with adequate therapy.	Acute coronary syndrome accompanied by myocardial tissue infarction. No ST elevation because there is no complete transmural ischaemia, either because of the absence of complete occlusion or the presence of collateral circulation.	Acute coronary syndrome in which there is myocardial tissue infarction. Transmural ischaemia occurs due to coronary artery occlusion, resulting in ST elevation. The infarction location in the heart depends on which coronary artery is occluded (see Figure 19).
E	Exact prevalence unknown	Incidence of acute myocardial infarction ♂ 2030:100,000 per y, ♀ 810:100,000 per y	
Ae	Unstable plaque rupture or erosion → activation of coagulation cascade → partial/total intraluminal occlusion → sharp decrease in coronary blood flow → ischaemia	Unstable plaque rupture or erosion → activation of coagulation cascade → partial/total intraluminal occlusion → sharp decrease in coronary blood flow → infarction → necrosis	Unstable plaque rupture or erosion → activation of coagulation cascade → complete coronary artery occlusion → transmural ischaemia with necrosis → ST elevation
R	General cardiovascular risk factors		
Hx	• Asymptomatic (25%) • Crushing CP, possibly radiating to left shoulder/arm and/or throat, dyspnoea on exertion, nausea, sweating		
PE	Anxious, sweaty, no increase of chest pain with palpitations, possibly subfebrile. S3 and S4 possibly audible upon auscultation.		
Dx	• Echocardiography: normal or hypokinesia/akinesia in the ischaemic area • CT coronary angiogram (CTCA) can be considered in case of normal troponin and ECG: quantification of coronary calcium score and coronary stenosis		
	Labs: troponins/CK-MB =	Labs: troponins/CK-MB ↑	

Table 68A // Acute coronary syndrome

<table>
<tr><th></th><th>UNSTABLE ANGINA PECTORIS</th><th>NON-ST ELEVATION MYOCARDIAL INFARCTION (NSTEMI)</th><th>ST ELEVATION MYOCARDIAL INFARCTION (STEMI)</th></tr>
<tr><td>Dx</td><td colspan="2">• 12-lead ECG: normal or ST depression/T-wave inversion
• CAG: normal or coronary stenoses</td><td>• ECG: ST elevations at presentation (see Figure 19 for ECG evolution and Table 29 for the localisation of ECG abnormalities)
• Coronary angiography: complete coronary occlusion</td></tr>
<tr><td rowspan="2">Tx</td><td colspan="3">• Continuous ECG monitoring, O_2 at SpO_2 <90%
• Acute phase: nitroglycerin and possibly morphine, loading dose of acetylsalicylic acid and P2Y12 inhibitor
• Post-acute phase: acetylsalicylic acid, P2Y12 inhibitor, statin, beta blocker, ACE inhibitor ('Golden five')
• Long-term: treat cardiac risk factors, lifestyle advice, cardiac rehabilitation
• Post-PCI: DAPT is recommended</td></tr>
<tr><td colspan="2">Abnormal CAG or cardiogenic shock:
• PCI
• CABG: in triple vessel disease, main coronary artery stenosis and combined valvular heart disease</td><td>Urgent revascularisation (<120 min): PCI or CABG. If PCI is not possible <120 min, thrombolysis should be considered.</td></tr>
<tr><td>P</td><td>May evolve into infarction with inadequate therapy</td><td colspan="2">• In-hospital mortality 4-12%
• Major cause of death worldwide</td></tr>
<tr><td>!</td><td>N/A</td><td colspan="2">• Acute complications (1-4d post-infarction): ventricular arrhythmias (fibrillation, tachycardias), bundle branch block, papillary muscle rupture, free wall rupture, ventricular septal defect, cardiogenic shock, HF
• Late complications: ventricular aneurysm, ischaemic cardiomyopathy, HF
• RV infarction is characterised by hypotension, distended neck veins, and clear lung auscultation. It is mostly associated with inferior and posterior LV infarction infarction and proximal RCA occlusion.</td></tr>
</table>

Table 68B // Acute coronary syndrome

Not all regions of the heart are sufficiently visualised in a standard 12-lead ECG. An isolated posterior STEMI can be seen as isolated ST depressions in V1-V3 as they mirror ST elevations over the posterior wall. Alternatively, the posterior wall can be visualised by adding dorsal leads V7-V9. Right-sided leads (V3R and V4R) can identify right ventricular involvement.

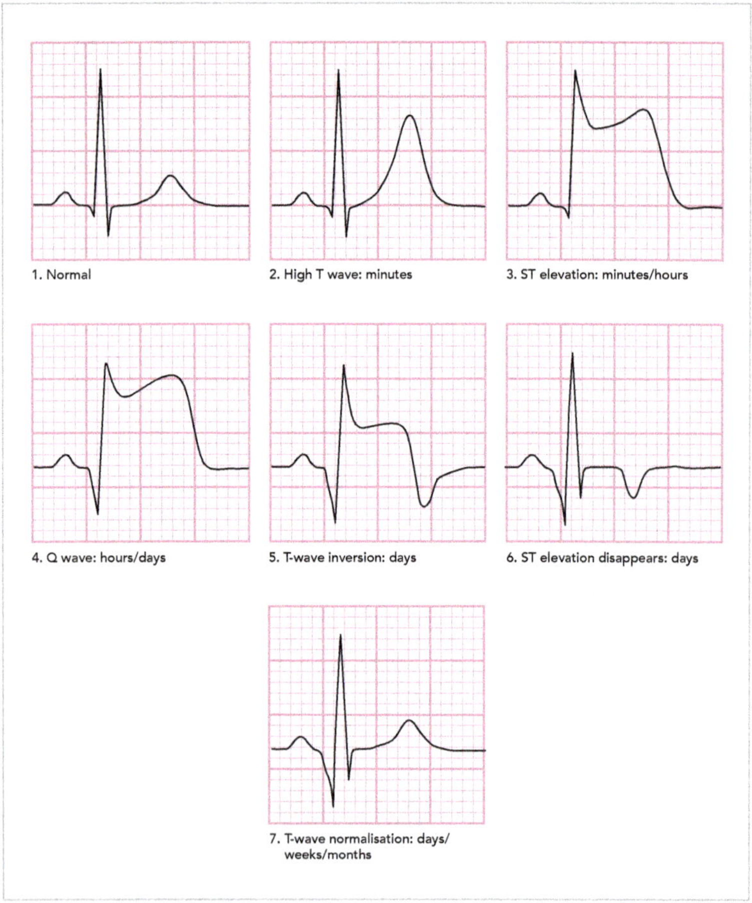

Figure 19 // ECG progression over time in infarction

Arrhythmia

D Arrhythmia is an abnormal cardiac rhythm that can range from harmless extrasystoles to life-threatening situations such as ventricular fibrillation. Arrhythmias are divided into supraventricular (atrial and AV-nodal) arrhythmias and ventricular arrhythmias. See Table 69 for the classification of heart rates.

Ae
- Abnormal impulse formation: abnormal automaticity, triggered activity
- Abnormal impulse conduction: re-entry

R Structural and ischaemic heart disease (++), hypertension, cardiac surgery, external factors (stress, fever, anaemia, hyperthyroidism, intoxications), positive family history (FHx)

Hx Asymptomatic, palpitations (frequency, regularity, continuous or episodic, concomitant symptoms, medication, provoking factors), fatigue, dizziness, syncope, CP, dyspnoea

PE Abnormal heart rate, regularity and/or pulse wave, watch for signs of HF (see Heart failure)

Dx
- Labs to rule out underlying pathology: hyperthyroidism, electrolyte disturbances, impaired glucose regulation, infection, intoxication. Consider urinary metanephrines for exclusion of pheochromocytoma.
- ECG and/or Holter monitoring: diagnosis of arrhythmias
- Echocardiography: diagnosis of underlying heart muscle or valve disease
- Stress test: diagnosis of stress-dependent arrhythmias
- Electrophysiological examination: diagnosis of the origin of arrhythmias

! Watch out for sudden cardiac arrest

FREQUENCY	RATE
Normal frequency	60-100/min
Bradycardia	<60/min
Tachycardia	>100/min

Table 69 // Heart rate terminology

AV block

D An AV block is a conduction disorder in which the AV node conducts impulses from the atria to the ventricles too slowly or not at all (see Table 70 and Figure 20).

> Second-degree type I AV block (Wenckebach) at night may be physiological, especially in adolescents and elite athletes.

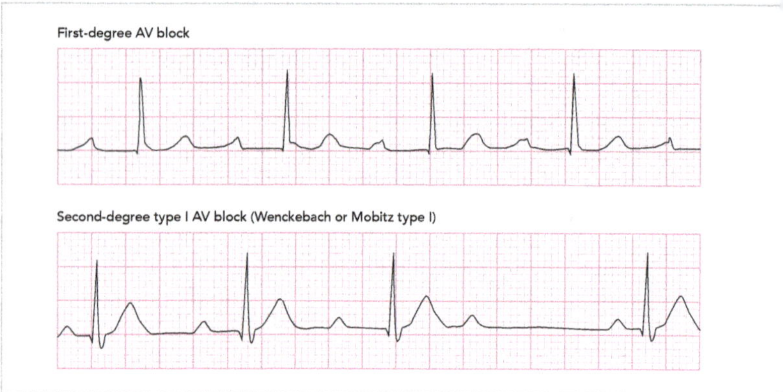

Figure 20 // Types of AV block

FEATURES	FIRST-DEGREE AV BLOCK	SECOND-DEGREE TYPE I AV BLOCK/WENCKEBACH
PQ INTERVAL	PQ interval >200 ms, each P wave is followed by a QRS complex	Gradual PQ interval ↑ until impulses from the atria are no longer conducted to the ventricles
Ae	Advanced age, medications (antiarrhythmics), AV node damage due to ischaemia, congenital, cardiac surgery or ablation procedures	Advanced age, medications (antiarrhythmics), AV node damage due to ischaemia, congenital, cardiac surgery or ablation procedures
Hx	Asymptomatic	Asymptomatic (++), dizziness, (pre-)syncope
Tx	Wait-and-see	Wait-and-see

Table 70 // Types of AV block

Supraventricular arrhythmias

- **The goal of rhythm control** is to restore sinus rhythm.
- **The goal of rate control** is to keep the ventricular rate <110/min and improve exercise tolerance.

Second-degree type II AV block (Mobitz type II)

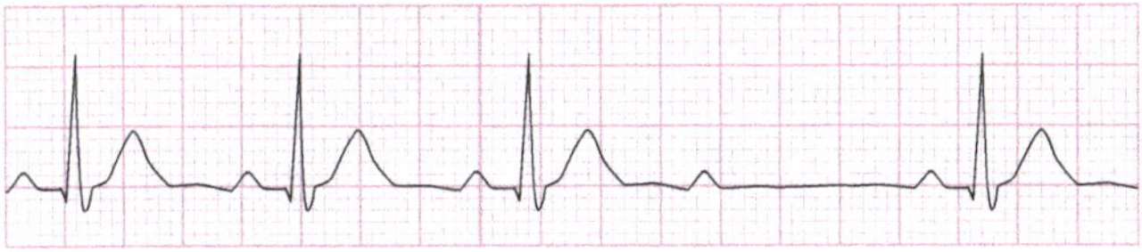

Third-degree (complete) AV block

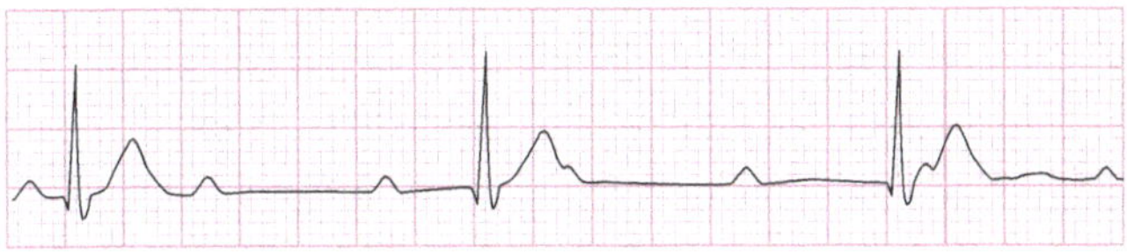

<table>
<tr><th>SECOND-DEGREE TYPE II AV BLOCK/ MOBITZ TYPE II</th><th>THIRD-DEGREE AV BLOCK</th></tr>
<tr><td>Sudden failure of impulse conduction from the atria to the ventricles, PQ interval remains constant (either normal or prolonged)</td><td>No impulse conduction from the atria to the ventricles (AV dissociation). Frequently results in a ventricular escape rhythm of 50/min. Atria and ventricles contract fully independently, both at their own constant rate.</td></tr>
<tr><td colspan="2">Advanced age, medications (antiarrhythmics), AV node damage due to ischaemia, congenital, cardiac surgery (transcatheter aortic valve implantation (TAVI)), or ablation procedures</td></tr>
<tr><td colspan="2">(Pre-)syncope, dizziness, fatigue, CP, sudden cardiac arrest</td></tr>
<tr><td colspan="2">Haemodynamically unstable: isoprenaline, atropine
Pacemaker</td></tr>
</table>

AF aetiologies: **PIRATES**

- **P**ulmonary conditions, **p**ostoperative
- **I**schaemic heart disease, **i**diopathic, **i**nfection
- **R**heumatic valve disease (mitral stenosis or regurgitation)
- **A**naemia, **a**lcohol, **a**ge, **a**utonomic
- **T**hyroid defects
- **E**levated BP (hypertension), **e**lectrocution
- **S**leep apnoea, **s**epsis, **s**urgery

<table>
<tr><th>FEATURES</th><th>ATRIAL FIBRILLATION</th><th>ATRIAL FLUTTER</th><th>ATRIAL TACHYCARDIA</th></tr>
<tr><td>REGULARITY</td><td>Irregular</td><td colspan="2">Regular</td></tr>
<tr><td>ATRIAL RATE</td><td>400-600/min</td><td>250-350/min</td><td>120-250/min</td></tr>
<tr><td>VENTRICULAR RATE</td><td>75-175/min</td><td>100/min in 3:1 AV block,
150/min in 2:1 AV block</td><td>75-200/min</td></tr>
<tr><td>ORIGIN</td><td>Atria (usually around the pulmonary veins)</td><td>Atria (re-entry circuits usually occur in the RA)</td><td>Atria</td></tr>
<tr><td>E</td><td>• Most common arrhythmia
• Incidence and prevalence increase with age, prevalence = 1% and prevalence at age ≥80 = 9% in the US.</td><td>Incidence and prevalence increase with age, prevalence ♂ 125:100,000, ♀ 59:100,000</td><td>• Prevalence: 0.3-0.5%
• Third most common paroxysmal SVT (10%)
• Mostly in middle age</td></tr>
<tr><td rowspan="2">Ae</td><td colspan="2">Hypertension</td><td rowspan="2">Cardiac ischaemia, sympathetic excitation, atrial overload, idiopathic</td></tr>
<tr><td>DM, obesity, HF, cardiomyopathy, valvular heart disease, congenital heart disease, ischaemic heart disease, hyperthyroidism, inflammation, fever, anaemia, COPD, alcohol</td><td>Congenital heart defects, after myocardial infarction or heart surgery, thyroid disease or lung disease</td></tr>
<tr><td>Hx</td><td colspan="3">Asymptomatic, palpitations (frequency, regularity (continuous or episodic)), concomitant symptoms, medication, provoking factors, fatigue, dizziness, loss of consciousness, CP, dyspnoea</td></tr>
<tr><td rowspan="2">PE</td><td colspan="3">• Abnormal heart rate, regularity and/or pulse wave
• Watch for signs of HF (see Heart failure)</td></tr>
<tr><td>Heart rate =/↑, irregular/normal, unequal/normal/pulse deficit</td><td colspan="2">Heart rate =/↑, regular</td></tr>
<tr><td>Dx</td><td colspan="3">• Labs to rule out underlying pathology: hyperthyroidism, electrolyte disturbances, impaired glucose regulation, infection, intoxication
• ECG and/or Holter monitor
• Transthoracic echocardiography
• Stress test: to diagnose stress-dependent arrhythmias
• Electrophysiological examination: to diagnose the origin of arrhythmias
• Cardiac computed tomography angiography (CCTA) in case of suspected CAD
• Consider TTE and cardiac MRI to identify underlying heart disease</td></tr>
</table>

Table 71A // Supraventricular tachycardias

AV RE-ENTRY TACHYCARDIA (AVRT)	AV NODAL RE-ENTRY TACHYCARDIA (AVNRT)	AV-JUNCTIONAL TACHYCARDIA
Regular		
150-250/min	100-280/min	60-100/min 70-130/min
Re-entry into the AV node and AV accessory bundle	Re-entry into the AV node	Increased automaticity of the AV node
• Second most common paroxysmal SVT (30%) • ♀>♂, mostly in childhood	• Most common paroxysmal SVT (50-60%) • ♀>♂, presents mostly in young adulthood	167:100,000 patients with heart disease age >65
Congenital accessory AV junction (bundle of Kent/Wolff-Parkinson-White syndrome)	Anterograde conduction down the 'slow' pathway and retrograde conduction down the 'fast' pathway in the AV node	Digoxin poisoning, myocardial infarction, after cardiac surgery, myocarditis
Asymptomatic, palpitations (frequency, regularity (continuous or episodic)), concomitant symptoms, medication, provoking factors, fatigue, dizziness, loss of consciousness, CP, dyspnoea		
• Abnormal heart rate, regularity and/or pulse wave, heart sounds, murmurs • Watch for signs of HF (see Heart failure)		
Heart rate =/↑, regular		
• Labs to rule out underlying pathology: hyperthyroidism, electrolyte disturbances, impaired glucose regulation, infection, intoxication • ECG and/or Holter monitor • Echocardiography: to rule out underlying heart disease • Stress test: to diagnose underlying heart muscle disease • Electrophysiological examination: to diagnose the origin of arrhythmias		

FEATURES	ATRIAL FIBRILLATION	ATRIAL FLUTTER	ATRIAL TACHYCARDIA
Tx	Acute: • Pharmacological cardioversion: antiarrhythmics (class I and III) • Anticoagulation if CHA_2DS_2-VA >1 • Rate control: beta blocker or digoxin Electric cardioversion (if AF >48h, 3 wk adequate anticoagulation therapy first) Post-acute: Educate patients to optimize shared decision-making • Rhythm control: antiarrhythmics (class I and III) • Rate control: beta blocker, diltiazem, digoxin • Anticoagulation start if CHA_2DS_2-VA ≥2 or comorbidity of hypertrophic cardiomyopathy or cardiac amyloidosis, consider if CHA_2DS_2-VA is 1 (see Table 75): DOAC, VKA (INR range 2.0-3.0) Ablation: pulmonary vein isolation in AF or cavotricuspid isthmus ablation in atrial flutter		Acute: Pharmacological cardioversion: class I antiarrhythmics • Beta blocker, diltiazem, amiodarone Electric cardioversion Post-acute: Antiarrhythmics: class I Ablation
!	• Risk of TIA/stroke and HF • AF can progress to atrial flutter and vice versa • Various types of AF (see Table 73)		N/A

Table 71B // Supraventricular tachycardias

FEATURES	SINUS BRADYCARDIA	SINUS ARREST
D	Sinus rhythm <60/min	No P waves on ECG for >2 sec
RATE	<60/min	Depends on escape rhythm
ORIGIN	Sinus node	
Ae	Vagus nerve stimulation ↑, sleep, hypothermia, hypoglycaemia, hypoxia, beta blocker	Vagus nerve stimulation ↑, sick sinus syndrome, drug-induced (lithium, digoxin, beta blockers), fibrosing sinus node
Tx	Treat underlying cause if necessary Stop negative chronotropic medication (beta blockers) Pacemaker	

Table 72 // Supraventricular bradycardias

AF SHAPE	DESCRIPTION
Paroxysmal	AF episodes that spontaneously convert to sinus rhythm <7d
Persistent	AF persisting >7d
Permanent	AF persisting >7d, with both patient and physician accepting the arrythmia. No further cardioversion is attempted.

Table 73 // Types of AF

<table>
<tr><th>AV RE-ENTRY TACHYCARDIA (AVRT)</th><th>AV NODAL RE-ENTRY TACHYCARDIA (AVNRT)</th><th>AV-JUNCTIONAL TACHYCARDIA</th></tr>
<tr><td colspan="2">Acute:
Modified, Vasalva manoeuvre
Pharmacological cardioversion: antiarrhythmics (class I - IV), adenosine
Electric cardioversion
Post-acute:
Antiarrhythmics: class I - IV, digoxin, non-dihydropiridines
Ablation (preferred treatment option)</td><td>Antiarrhythmics (class I, II and III)</td></tr>
<tr><td>N/A</td><td>Risk of AV block for which <1% require a pacemaker</td><td>N/A</td></tr>
</table>

Sick sinus syndrome

D Sick sinus syndrome is an umbrella term for conditions arising from sinus node dysfunction. This syndrome can lead to sinus bradycardia, sinus arrest and supraventricular tachycardia. ECG abnormalities must be related to symptoms. Escape rhythms can take over (see Table 74 and Figure 21).

E Incidence 100:100,000 per year

Ae Idiopathic degeneration of sinus node cells, autonomic dysfunction, damaged myocardium due to ischaemia or surgery, drug-induced (beta blockers, calcium channel blockers, antiarrhythmics, digoxin), infectious, paraneoplastic, cardiomyopathy

R Age >65, systemic disease, ischaemic heart disease, structural heart disease

Hx Asymptomatic, hot flashes, (pre-) syncope, fatigue, dyspnoea, palpitations

PE No specific findings, BP, oedema, heart sounds, murmurs and signs of systemic disease

Dx
- ECG and/or Holter monitoring: sinus bradycardia, sinus arrest, escape rhythms, SVT
- Echocardiography: to show/rule out underlying heart defects

Tx Wait-and-see if asymptomatic

- Drug interventions are only of possible use in acute situations (atropine, isoprenaline)
- Pacemaker

Ⓟ Complications: atrial fibrillation or total AV block

EVENT	ATRIAL ESCAPE RHYTHM	JUNCTIONAL ESCAPE RHYTHM	VENTRICULAR ESCAPE RHYTHM
ECG characteristics	Narrow QRS complex, abnormal P wave morphology	Narrow QRS complex, AV dissociation	Wide QRS complex, AV dissociation
Atrial rate	60-80/min	40-60/min	20-40/min
Origin	Atria	AV node	Ventricles

Table 74 // Escape rhythms

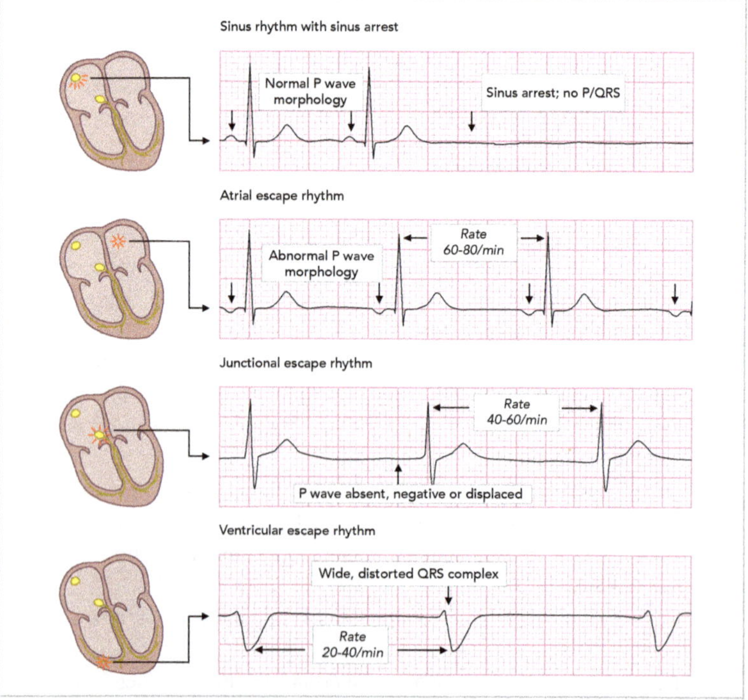

Figure 21 // Escape rhythms

SYMBOL	MEANING	SCORE
C	Congestive HF	1
H	Hypertension	1
A_2	Age ≥75	2
D	DM	1
S_2	Stroke/TIA/arterial thromboembolism	2
V	Vascular disease	1
A	Age 65-74	1

Table 75 // CHA_2DS_2-VA score

Ventricular arrhythmias

Ventricular arrhythmia

D Ventricular arrhythmias originate in the ventricles, and occur when the heart is excited not by the conduction system but by cardiomyocytes, resulting in broad QRS complexes on ECG (see Tables 76 and 77 and Figure 22).

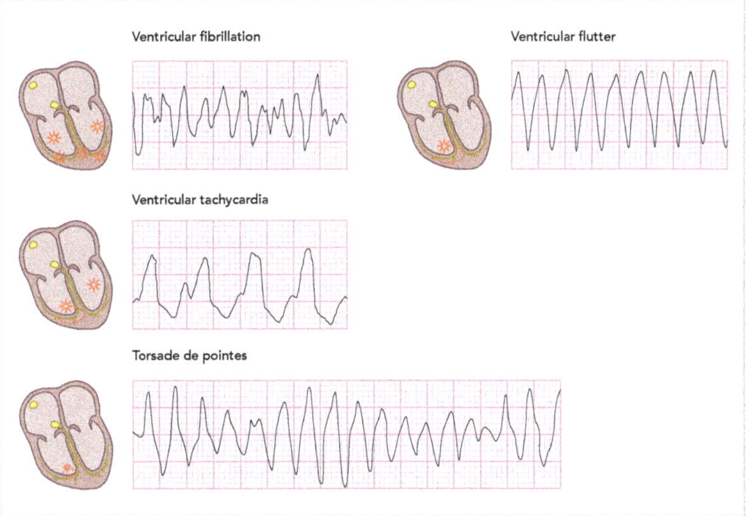

Figure 22 // Ventricular tachycardias

FEATURES	VENTRICULAR FIBRILLATION	VENTRICULAR FLUTTER
REGULARITY	Irregular	Regular
ATRIAL RATE	60-100/min	
VENTRICULAR RATE	400-600/min	150-300/min
Ae	• Clusters of ventricular cardiomyocytes fire spontaneously → ineffective ventricular pumping function • Frequently occurs <48h after myocardial infarction	Re-entry circuit → ineffective ventricular pumping function
Tx	CPR Defibrillation	• Acute: cardioversion • Post-acute: ablation

Table 76 // Ventricular arrhythmias

VENTRICULAR TACHYCARDIA	DEFINITION
Non-sustained VT	≥3 ventricular beats with a max. duration of 30 sec
Sustained VT	VT lasts >30 sec or is symptomatic
Monomorphic VT	All ventricular beats are uniform
Polymorphic VT	• Beat-to-beat variation between ventricular beats • Watch out: high risk of progressing to ventricular fibrillation
Biphasic VT	• Complex-to-complex variation between ventricular beats • Watch out: associated with long QT syndrome and digoxin poisoning

Table 77 // Ventricular tachycardias

Bundle branch block (BBB)

D A BBB is a conduction disorder in which impulse conduction by the bundle branches slows down or ceases. In right bundle branch block (RBBB), impulse conduction across the right bundle branch slows down or ceases. In left bundle branch block (LBBB) the same happens across the left bundle branch. Characteristic ECG findings for BBB are a widened QRS. With an incom-

VENTRICULAR TACHYCARDIA	TORSADE DE POINTES
Regular	
60-100/min	
110-250/min	150-300/min
• Ventricular ectopic focus or re-entry firing at a rate >100/min, dominating the sinus rhythm • For classification, see Table 76	QT interval ↑ combined with micro re-entry circuit in ventricle → QRS complexes circulate around baseline
Acute: Cardioversion Post-acute: Antiarrhythmics Ablation, ICD	Treat underlying cause • Stop provoking drugs • Correct electrolyte disorders • Medication: beta blockers, antiarrhythmics • Acute situation: magnesium IV ICD

plete block, QRS interval 100-120 ms. With a complete block, QRS interval ≥120 ms (see Table 78).

Tx In HF with reduced ejection fraction (HFrEF) and BBB, consider a biventricular pacemaker or ICD

ITEM	RIGHT BUNDLE BRANCH BLOCK (RBBB)	LEFT BUNDLE BRANCH BLOCK (LBBB)	LEFT ANTERIOR HEMIBLOCK	LEFT POSTERIOR HEMIBLOCK
Blocked branch	Right bundle branch	Left bundle branch	Anterior bundle of the left bundle branch	Posterior bundle of the left bundle branch
Characteristics	• RSR' (rabbit ears) in V1 • Wide S in I, aVL, V6	• QS or RS in V1 • Wide R and no Q in I, aVL, V6	• Left axis deviation • S>R in II, III, and aVF, and slow R wave progression in precordial leads • Small S in I and aVL (see Figure 24)	• Right axis deviation • Deep S in I and aVL • Small Q in III and aVF (see Figure 24)
QRS duration	≥120 ms		100-120 ms	
Aetiology	RV overload, cardiomyopathy, ischaemia, aging	Cardiomyopathy, ischaemia, hypertension	Cardiac ischaemia, hypertension, cardiomyopathy, aortic valve defects, connective tissue disease	

Table 78 // Bundle branch block

In RBBB, the QRS complex in V1 resembles rabbit ears on ECG. In LBBB, the QRS complex in V1 resembles a bag of French fries (See Figure 23).

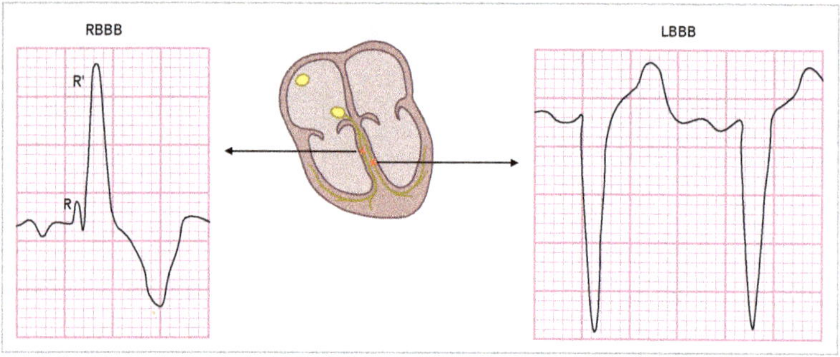

Figure 23 // Left and right bundle branch block in lead V1

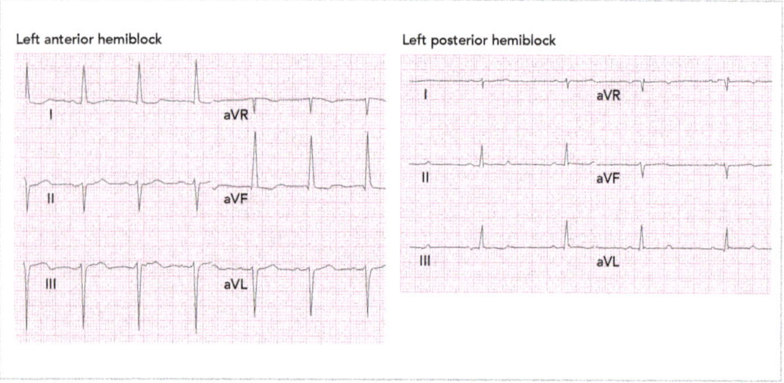

Figure 24 // ECG showing left anterior hemiblock and left posterior hemiblock

Endocarditis

Infective endocarditis (IE)

D IE is an acute or subacute microbial inflammation of the endocardium and valves or of an intracardiac device. Acute IE usually involves a native valve and is often accompanied by metastatic foci of infection. Subacute endocarditis often involves a damaged heart valve and metastatic abscesses are rare. The clinical diagnosis of endocarditis is made using the modified Duke criteria (see Table 79). The diagnosis of definite endocarditis must meet **1** two major criteria, **2** one major criterion and three minor criteria, or **3** five minor criteria. A diagnosis of possible endocarditis must meet **1** one major criterion and one minor criterion or **2** three minor criteria.

E Incidence 5-35:100,000 per year

Ae Typical pathogens: Staphylococcus aureus (acute IE), Streptococcus viridans, enterococci (subacute IE), Streptococcus gallolyticus (Streptococcus bovis), HACEK (Haemophilus species, Aggregatibacter actinomycetemcomitans, Cardiobacterium hominis, Eikenella corrodens, Kingella kingae) group

R Age >60, ♂, artificial valve or stent, congenital and structural heart defects, dental surgery, IV drug use, chronic haemodialysis, PMHx: endocarditis

Hx Fever (90%), malaise, arthralgia, back pain

PE T ↑, splinter haemorrhages under the nails (see Figure 25), Janeway lesions (see Figure 26), Osler nodules, murmur (85%, location depends on affected valve), throbbing spine, focal neurological abnormalities in septic emboli

Dx
- Labs: CRP ↑, BSE ↑, WBC ↑, lactate dehydrogenase ↑ (in haemolysis)
- Urine: microscopic haematuria
- Blood cultures +
- Echocardiography (reference standard is transoesophageal echocardiography (TOE)): vegetations (see Figure 27), abscesses, pseudoaneurysms, intracardiac fistulae, valve perforation, new partial dehiscence of artificial valve
- For strong suspicion of IE but negative TOE: brain MRI/spleen MRI/PET-CT/SPECT-CT

Tx
- AB IV for 4-6 wk depending on the microorganism, frequently with >1 medication initially
- In ±50% of patients, valve replacement and/or surgical removal of infected material or abscesses, including artificial material and devices such as a pacemaker or artificial valve. Early surgery is recommended with complications or risk of complications.

P
- Mortality: 15-30%
- Depends on the condition of the patient and the microorganism involved. Poor in cases of HF, periannular complications and/or Staphylococcus aureus infection.

I Risk of HF, septic shock, valvular heart disease, embolic complications (brain, spleen, extremities), abscess formation, infectious aneurysms, myocarditis and pericarditis, acute renal failure, arrhythmias

In patients presenting with embolic complications and fever with unknown aetiology, always consider endocarditis. Approx. 25% of patients have embolic complications at the time of diagnosis.

- **Janeway lesions:** non-painful, erythematous macules/nodules a few mm in size mainly on palms and soles of feet.
- **Osler nodules:** painful, erythematous nodules a few mm in size mainly on fingers and toes.

MAJOR CRITERIA	MINOR CRITERIA
Positive blood cultures: • Typical microorganisms for IE from two separate blood cultures: - Streptococcus viridans, Streptococcus gallolyticus (Streptococcus bovis), HACEK group, Staphylococcus aureus - Community-acquired enterococci in the absence of a primary focus • Microorganisms consistent with IE from persistently positive blood cultures: - ≥2 blood cultures taken >12h apart - All three or the majority of ≥4 different blood cultures (with >1h between the first and last blood culture) • 1 blood culture with Coxiella burnetii or IgG antibody titre >1:800 Positive imaging: • Positive echocardiography: vegetations, abscess/pseudoaneurysms/intracardiac fistula, valve perforation/aneurysms, new partial dehiscence of the artificial valve • Abnormal activity around artificial valve on PET-CT or SPECT-CT • Paravalvular lesions on cardiac CT	• Predisposing cardiac lesion, see risk factors • T ≥38°C • Vascular phenomena: arterial embolisms, septic pulmonary infarctions, mycotic aneurysms, intracranial haemorrhage, conjunctival haemorrhage, Janeway lesions • Immunologic phenomena: glomerulonephritis, Osler nodules, splinter haemorrhages, positive rheumatoid factor • Microbiological evidence: - Positive blood cultures that do not meet a major criterion - Serological evidence of active infection with an organism consistent with IE

Table 79 // Modified Duke criteria for the diagnosis of infective endocarditis

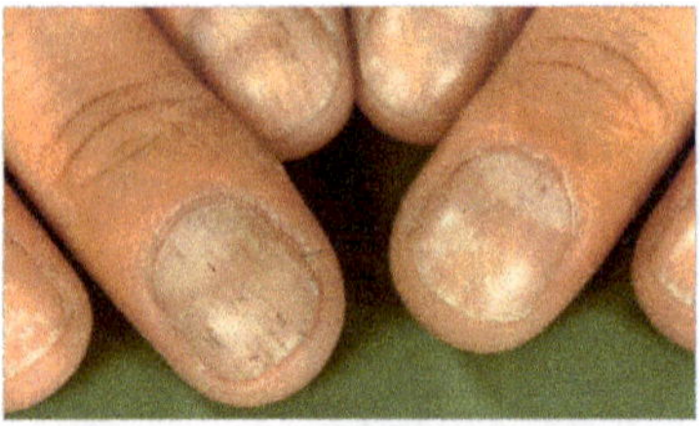

Figure 25 // Splinter haemorrhages under the nails

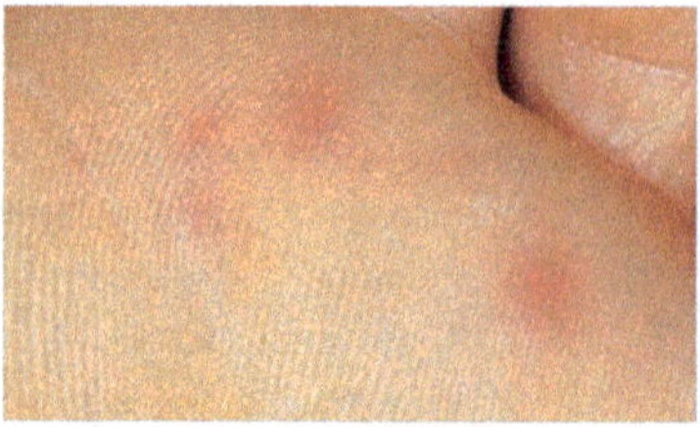

Figure 26 // Janeway lesions

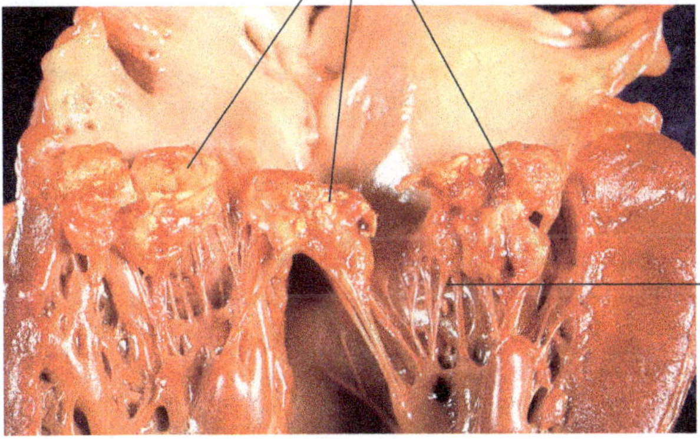

Figure 27 // Post-mortem vegetations on mitral valve

Heart failure (HF)

Heart failure (HF)

D HF, also called congestive heart failure, is a clinical syndrome caused by functional or structural cardiac pathology that results in decreased CO and/or increased intracardiac pressure. A distinction is made between chronic HF with preserved ejection fraction (HFpEF), with mildly reduced ejection fraction (HFmrEF) and with reduced ejection fraction (HFrEF), and acute HF (see Table 80).

E Prevalence in adult population = 1-2%, prevalence at age ≥70 = 10% and at age ≥85 = 20%

Ae Systolic function ↓, diastolic function ↓

R General cardiovascular risk factors (see Table 80)

Hx See Table 80 and Figure 28

PE See Table 80 and Figure 28

Dx
- Labs: NT-proBNP or other natriuretic peptides ↑
- ECG: possibly information about aetiology. HF is unlikely with a normal ECG.
- Chest X-ray to rule out pulmonary pathology: signs of acute HF
- Echocardiography (gold standard): information about aetiology and cardiac function

- Cardiac MRI/PET-CT/CTCA/cardiac catheterisation (if ultrasound is inconclusive): information about aetiology, atrial and ventricular pressure and cardiac function
- Stress ultrasound or ECG (in follow-up phase): evaluation of exercise capacity

Tx
- Treat underlying cause
- Treatment is aimed at reducing symptoms, maintaining quality of life and improving prognosis
- Smoking cessation (especially with underlying coronary artery disease), exercise ↑, weight reduction, dietary changes (saturated fats/carbohydrates/salt/caffeine ↓, unsaturated fats ↑, fruit/vegetables ↑, fluid restriction), avoid alcohol consumption, avoid stress

See Table 80

P
- Depending on underlying cause, comorbidities and overall condition of patient
- 1-year mortality after hospitalisation (largely independent of aetiology): ±17%, in stable patients: ±7%

! Risk of cardiogenic shock, progression of HF and sudden cardiac arrest

HF can be categorised in several ways, with HFpEF and HFrEF being the most commonly used classifiers. Other ways to categorise HF include:

- Left-sided vs. right-sided HF (see Figure 28): HFpEF and HFrEF are types of left-sided HF with impaired LV diastolic function/output. Right-sided HF involves impaired RV diastolic function/output. Right-sided HF frequently results from left-sided HF, chronic pulmonary disease, or pulmonary hypertension. Symptoms and signs of fluid overload are the most evident indicators of right-sided HF, followed by shortness of breath.
- Diastolic vs. systolic HF: HFpEF and HfrEF have long been used for diastolic HF and systolic HF, respectively. Since HF frequently has both a diastolic and a systolic component, these two terms provide greater accuracy.

HF is an unlikely diagnosis with completely normal NT-proBNP levels. Even elevated NT-proBNP levels may not always indicate HF, as other factors such as AF, renal failure and severe infections can also lead to an increase in NT-proBNP.

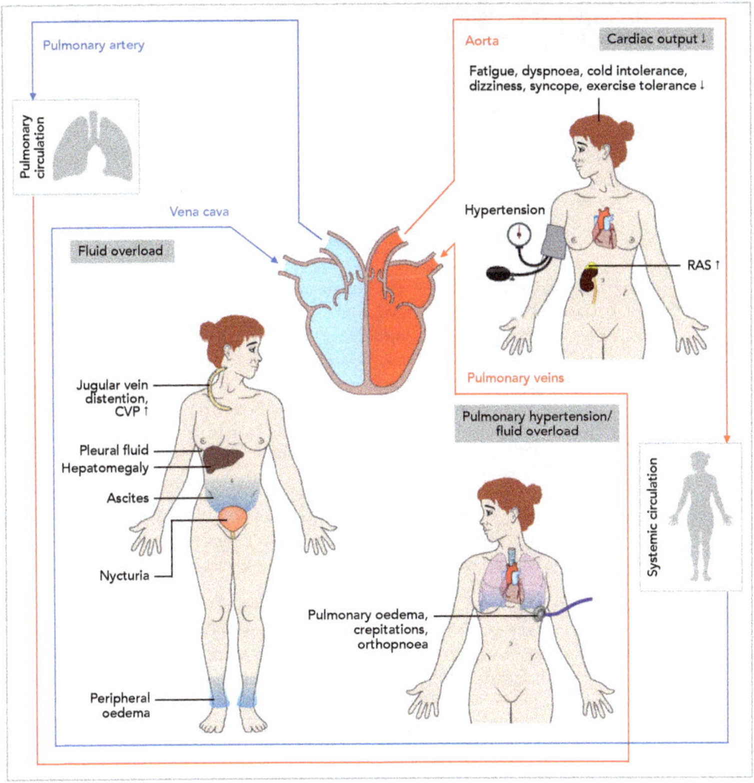

Figure 28 // Clinical symptoms of HF

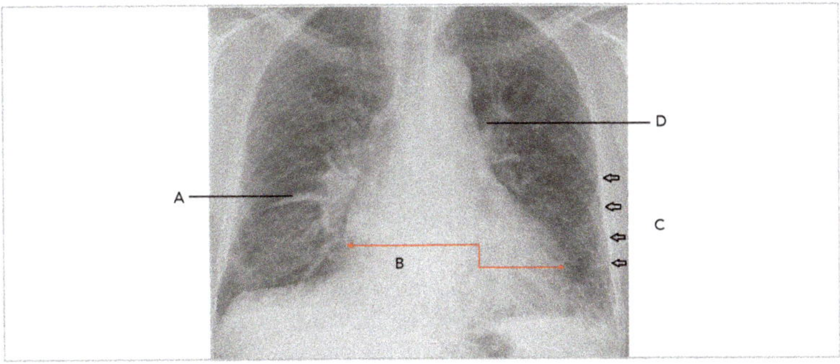

Figure 29 // Radiological characteristics of cardiac asthma on chest X-ray

A: Pleural fluid **B:** Cardiomegaly **C:** Kerley B lines **D:** Increased bronchovascular markings/redistribution

	HF WITH PRESERVED EJECTION FRACTION (HFpEF)	HF WITH REDUCED EJECTION FRACTION (HFrEF)
D	HF with left ventricular ejection fraction (LVEF) ≥50%, usually with normal LV volumes and evidence of diastolic dysfunction and/or structural heart disease.	HF with increased LV volumes and LVEF ≤40%.
E	HFpEF > HFrEF	
Ae	Ischaemic heart disease (⊕ with HFrEF), hypertension (⊕ with HFpEF), cardiomyopathies, valvular heart disease, arrhythmias, cardiac infections, congenital heart defects, metabolic abnormalities (including DM, obesity, thyroid abnormalities and hypercortisolism), renal failure, myocardial toxicity (e.g. substance abuse, heavy metal exposure, radiotherapy and medication such as cytostatics, antidepressants and antiarrhythmics), high output (e.g. sepsis, severe anaemia, pregnancy), cardiac neoplasms ⊖	
R	Age >60, ♀, hypertension, AF, COPD, DM, metabolic syndrome	PMHx: myocardial disease → hypokinesia
Hx	Dyspnoea on exertion ⊕, orthopnoea ⊕, nocturnal dyspnoea ⊕, bendopnoea (dyspnoea when leaning forward), exertional tolerance ↓ ⊕, fatigue ⊕, appetite ↓, nocturnal coughing, palpitations, dizziness, confusion, cold intolerance, syncope	
PE	• Inspection: CVP ↑ ⊕, weight ↑ (>2 kg/wk), weight ↓/cachexia (advanced HF) • Heart: S3 ⊕ in HFrEF and S4 ⊕ in HFpEF, apex beat palpable beyond midclavicular line ⊕, murmur (in case of valvular heart disease/endocarditis), heart rate ↑ • Pulmonary: pulmonary crepitations, attenuation of lower lung fields (with pleural fluid), basal breathing sound ↓ (with pleural fluid) • Miscellaneous: peripheral pitting oedema ⊕, hepatosplenomegaly, ascites, cold extremities (in hypoperfusion), oliguria (in hypoperfusion)	
Dx	Labs: NT-proBNP ↑, watch for signs of anaemia and monitor liver and kidney function regularly	
	Echocardiography and Doppler: LVEF ≥50%, LVH/concentric remodelling, LA enlargement, pulmonary artery pressure ↑, structural cardiac abnormalities	Echocardiography: LVEF <40%, often functional MR

Table 80A // Types of HF

> 40-49% of patients with an abnormal LVEF belong to the HFmrEF group. HFmrEF is a mild systolic dysfunction with features of diastolic dysfunction. These patients are likely to benefit from the same treatment as patients with HFrEF, but research is still ongoing.

ACUTE HF

Rapid onset or rapid increase in symptoms of HF, the most pronounced symptom usually being acute dyspnoea at rest/during minimal exertion. This may be an initial manifestation of HF or chronic decompensated HF.

- 15-20%: first manifestation of HF
- 70-80%: chronic decompensated HF

- Primary cardiac causes: ACS, arrhythmias/conduction disorders, acute valvular heart disease, acute mechanical aetiology (myocardial rupture, chest trauma, aortic dissection)
- Extrinsic factors: hypertensive emergency, pulmonary embolism, COPD exacerbation, infection, medication (NSAIDs, corticosteroids, negative inotropes), metabolic dysregulation (thyroid abnormalities, DKA, adrenal dysfunction), stroke, therapy noncompliance

Chronic HF

- In fluid overload at rest (95%): especially dyspnoea on exertion/orthopnoea/nighttime dyspnoea/bendopnoea
- In hypoperfusion: especially fatigue, dizziness, confusion, syncope

- Fluid overload at rest: normotensive-hypertensive, CVP ↑, peripheral oedema, pulmonary oedema/attenuation of lower lung fields, hepatosplenomegaly, ascites
- Hypoperfusion: hypotensive-normotensive, cold extremities, oliguria, consciousness ↓, low pulse pressure

Labs: NT-proBNP ↑, watch for signs of anaemia and monitor liver and kidney function regularly

- ECG: information about aetiology
- Chest X-ray: alveolar oedema, Kerley B lines, bronchovascular markings/redistribution ↑, pleural fluid (see Figure 29)
- Echocardiography: information about aetiology and cardiac function, evaluation of volume status (volume of inferior vena cava)
- In suspected pulmonary embolism: CT pulmonary angiogram

The severity of HF is determined using the **New York Heart Association (NYHA) classification** for HF:

- NYHA I: asymptomatic
- NYHA II: dyspnoea during strenuous exercise
- NYHA III: dyspnoea during moderate exercise
- NYHA IV: dyspnoea at rest or during mild exercise

	HF WITH PRESERVED EJECTION FRACTION (HFpEF)	HF WITH REDUCED EJECTION FRACTION (HFrEF)
Tx	Treat underlying cause and associated conditions (e.g. hypertension, DM, AF), lifestyle changes	
	• For signs of congestion: diuretics • Screening for/treatment of cardiovascular and non-cardiovascular comorbidities • SGLT-2 inhibitor Consider heart transplantation if above treatment options fail and patient reaches end-stage HF at age <65 in the absence of co-morbidities	In any patient with symptomatic HF: • ACE inhibitor or ARNI (angiotensin receptor neprilysin inhibitor), ARB in case of intolerance • Add beta blocker as soon as patient is clinically stable (no obvious fluid overload) • Aldosterone antagonist • SGLT2 inhibitor, e.g. dapagliflozin or empagliflozin In specific cases, consider: • Loop diuretic for congestion, possibly in conjunction with thiazide diuretic • Ivabradine for LVEF ≤35% if sinus rhythm and heart rate ≥75/min despite beta blocker therapy • Digoxin in AF for rate control • Consider ICD if LVEF ≤35% with ischaemic origin despite optimal therapy or symptomatic VF/VT in PMHx • If sinus rhythm and QRS ≥130 ms: consider cardiac resynchronisation therapy (CRT) • If the above treatment options fail: consider left ventricular assist device (LVAD)/heart transplantation
P	Mortality HFrEF > HFpEF	
!	Risk of acute HF/congestive HF	

Table 80B // Types of HF

Pericardial disease

Cardiac tamponade

D Cardiac tamponade is a medical emergency that takes place when abnormal amounts of fluid (e.g. blood, pus) accumulate in the pericardial sac, compressing the heart and leading to a decrease in cardiac output (CO). Cardiac tamponade is categorised by its origin: acute (minutes) or sub-acute (days/weeks).

E Incidence 50:100,000 hospital admissions

Ae Idiopathic, malignancy, pericarditis, sharp trauma, Dressler syndrome (post-myocardial infarction or post-cardiotomy)

R Autoimmune

ACUTE HF

Treat underlying cause/provoking factors

- In hypoxia: O_2 (max. saturation 98%)
- Loop diuretics IV, possibly in conjunction with thiazide diuretics/aldosterone antagonists to prevent hypokalaemia caused by loop diuretics
- Nitroglycerin IV: preload optimisation and afterload reduction
- If diuretics/vasodilators have insufficient effect/hypotensive effect: inotropes
- Avoid opiates (except in cases of severe dyspnoea/anxiety) due to risk of hypotension, bradycardia and respiratory depression

CHAMP

Most common causes of acute HF requiring prompt intervention:

C: acute **c**oronary syndrome
H: **h**ypertensive emergency
A: **a**rrhythmia
M: acute **m**echanical cause
P: **p**ulmonary embolism

30-day mortality: 5-10%, 1-year mortality: 20-40%

Risk of cardiogenic shock and sudden cardiac arrest

Hx
- Acute: dyspnoea, chest pain
- Sub-acute: dyspnoea, chest pain, fatigue

PE BP ↓, heart rate ↑, CVP ↑, paradoxical pulse, pericardial rub (a result of pericarditis), peripheral oedema

Dx
- ECG: microvoltages, QRS alternans
- Cardiac ultrasound: free fluid in the pericardium, collaps of RA and/or RV, widening of the IVC /widened IVC without collaps
- Lab: lactate ↑, creatinine ↑

Tx IV volume replacement as a temporary therapy before definitive treatment. Do not delay definitive pericardiocentesis treatment.

- Pericardiocentesis: percutaneous drainage of the pericardium to remove the obstruction

- Pericardiostomy: by means of thoracotomy and surgical opening of the pericardium to remove the obstruction

P In the case of traumatic cardiac tamponade: high mortality as a result of patient delay or diagnostic delay

! Beware of obstructive shock

> **Paradoxical pulse** occurs with cardiac tamponade, among other conditions. This phenomenon is characterised by an audible heart beat upon inhalation, but no palpable heart beat in the wrist. This is caused by an increase in negative intrathoracic pressure, which eventually results in decreased stroke volume and pulse amplitude, meaning that the heart beat is no longer palpable.

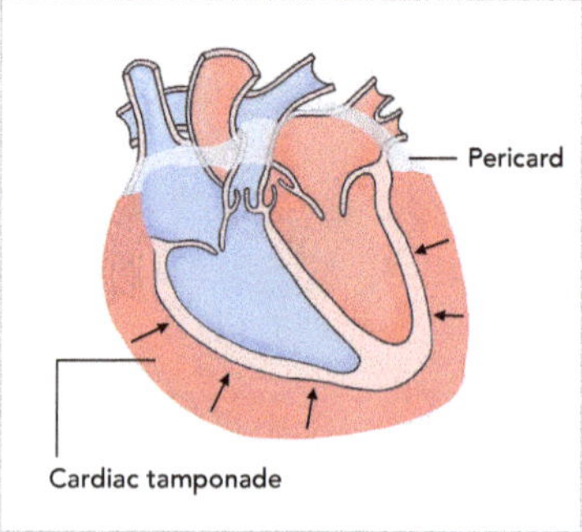

Figure 30 // Cardiac tamponade

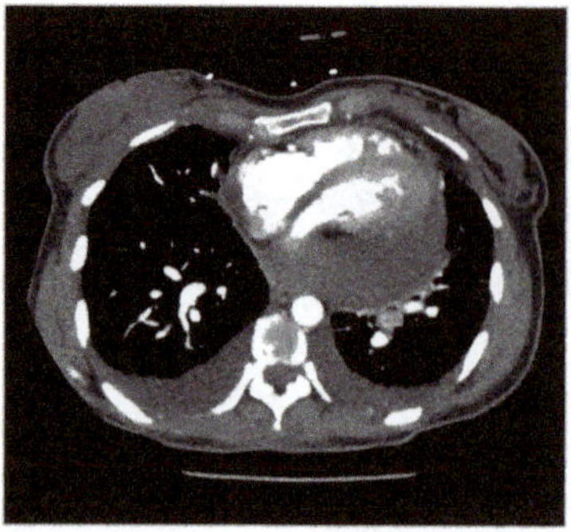

Figure 31 // CT image of cardiac tamponade showing pericardial fluid compressing the left ventricle.

Pericarditis

D Pericarditis is an inflammation of the pericardium and can occur in isolation or as part of local or systemic disease. Patients may present with acute pericarditis, chronic pericarditis or asymptomatic pericardial effusion.

E Incidence 28:100,000 per year, ±0.1% of all hospitalisations

Ae
- Idiopathic ⊕ (see Figure 32)
- Infectious: viral ⊕⊕ (after upper respiratory tract infection/gastroenteritis) or bacterial ⊖. For patients from low and middle income countries also consider HIV/tuberculosis.
- Autoimmune: including systemic lupus erythematosus (SLE), rheumatoid arthritis, IBD (inflammatory bowel disease)

- Malignancy: lung/breast cancer, Hodgkin lymphoma, mesothelioma
- Cardiac: cardiac surgery, post-myocardial infarction (Dressler's syndrome)
- Metabolic: uraemia, hypothyroidism

R Age 16-65, ♂, congenital heart defects

Hx Sharp chest pain, fever, general malaise, pain worsens when lying down/breathing in, pain improves in sitting/prone position

PE T ↑, auscultation: pericardial rub ⊖

Dx
- Labs: CRP ↑, BSE ↑, WBC ↑, troponin/CK-MB = (in pericardial myocarditis, cardiac enzymes may be elevated), test for underlying cause if indicated
- ECG: generalised concave ST elevation and PTa depression (acute phase) followed by negative T waves and finally normalisation
- Echocardiography: pericardial effusion, impaired pumping function (if perimyocarditis)
- Chest X-ray: CTR ↑ indicative for pericardial effusion, pulmonary oedema ⊖, armoured heart (i.e. calcified constrictive pericarditis) ⊖

Tx Treat underlying cause

Pain relief, anti-inflammatory therapy (NSAIDs, aspirin), colchicine to prevent recurrence, AB in bacterial infection ⊖

Pericardial fluid drainage for filling function ↓, partial removal of pericardium for constrictive pericarditis

P Good long-term prognosis, poor prognosis for high fever, subacute course, ample pericardial effusion and cardiac tamponade, 15-30% recurrence rate if not treated with colchicine

! Risk of cardiac tamponade, perimyocarditis, constrictive pericarditis ⊖

The typical patient with pericarditis is male, age 15-65, and presents with sharp CP that worsens with coughing and inhalation, improves when sitting upright and leaning forward, and is sometimes accompanied by fever. It typically starts a few days after flu-like symptoms.

Pericardial rub upon auscultation sounds like walking on fresh snow and can best be distinguished from pleural rub by asking the patient to hold their breath. Pleural rub will disappear, while pericardial rub will persist. Pericardial rub is easiest to hear in the left parasternal region.

≥2 major criteria for diagnosis of pericarditis:
- ECG abnormalities suited for pericarditis
- Pericardial rub
- Pericarditic chest pain
- Pericardial effusion

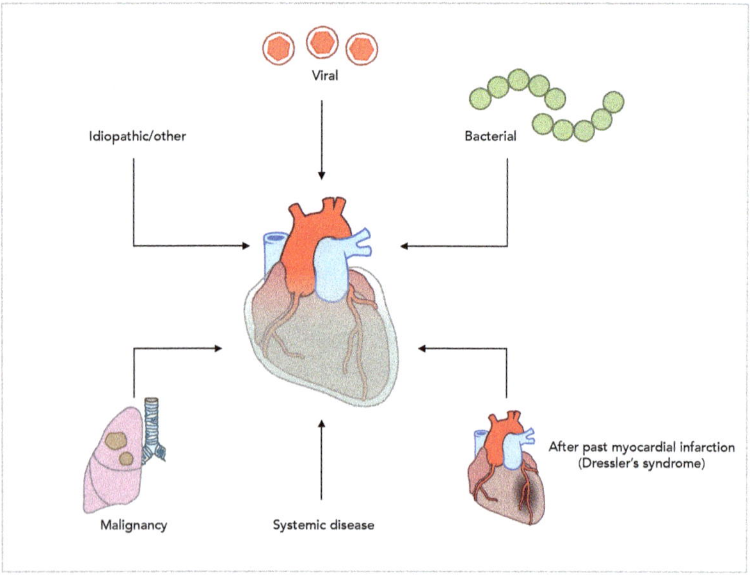

Figure 32 // Causes of pericarditis

Valvular heart disease

Valvular heart disease

D Valvular heart disease are characterised by impaired function of at least one heart valve, which may involve stenosis and/or regurgitation. See Table 81 for a list of valvular heart disease.

E Prevalence of moderate/severe valvular heart disease at age ≥75 = ±12.5%, aortic valve stenosis and mitral regurgitation are most common

Dx
- ECG: often nonspecific, sometimes atrial/ventricular enlargement/hypertrophy and/or arrhythmias
- Chest X-ray: cardiomegaly

- Echocardiography and Doppler (most-used diagnostic tool): abnormal valve shape and/or movement, severity of stenosis/regurgitation (Doppler), analyse cardiac function, indications of aetiology (including vegetations, annulus dilation)
- Cardiac MRI (if ultrasound is inconclusive): clear view of any abnormal valve morphology, ventricular function, severity of valvular heart disease (flow measurement, leak volume) and indications of aetiology
- ECG-triggered CT of the heart and aortic arch: accurate tool for detecting severity of valve calcification and abnormalities of ascending aorta in particular
- Cardiac catheterisation (if noninvasive tests are inconclusive): intracardiac pressure measurement, ventricular function, severity of valvular heart disease (for stenosis: pressure gradient across valve)
- Stress ultrasound/ECG: to evaluate exercise capacity in follow-up

Tx

- Conservative if minor valvular heart disease or poor surgical candidate (large number of comorbidities, limited life expectancy or poor cardiac function)
- Eliminate or treat underlying cause

Treat HF (see Heart failure)

- Valve repair or replacement with mechanical or bioprosthetic valve in severe, symptomatic valvular heart disease
- Percutaneous surgery in severe, symptomatic valvular heart disease and poor surgical candidates

The typical patient with aortic valve stenosis is age >75 and presents with CP, dyspnoea and/or syncope during exertion. During PE a systolic crescendo-decrescendo murmur is heard that radiates to the carotids and thoracic wall. Thrills can be felt along the jugular and in the neck.

The typical patient with mitral valve regurgitation is age >75 and presents with dyspnoea on exertion, fatigue and/or impaired exertional tolerance. During physical examination a holosystolic murmur is heard that radiates to the left armpit.

Systolic murmur:

- Aortic valve stenosis/pulmonary valve stenosis
- Mitral valve regurgitation/tricuspid valve regurgitation

Diastolic murmur:

- Aortic valve regurgitation/pulmonary valve regurgitation
- Mitral valve stenosis/tricuspid valve stenosis

Murmur intensity is scored on a scale of I-VI. A grade I murmur is barely audible with a stethoscope, while a grade VI murmur can be heard even without a stethoscope. Murmur intensity is not necessarily indicative of the severity of the abnormality.

	AORTIC VALVE REGURGITATION (AR)	AORTIC VALVE STENOSIS (AS)
D	Incomplete closure of the aortic valve, allowing blood to flow back to the LV during diastole and resulting in LV volume overload.	Incomplete opening of the aortic valve, leading to LV pressure overload.
E	Physiological AR is common in adults, prevalence at age 65-74 = 0.2%, prevalence at age >75 = 2%	Prevalence at age 65-74 = 1%, prevalence at age >75 = 3%
Ae	Degenerative (valvular calcification), infective endocarditis, acute rheumatoid arthritis, hypertension, congenital, aortic root disease (e.g. dilation, dissection of the ascending aorta), connective tissue disease, syphilis	Degenerative (valvular calcification ⊕), congenital (bicuspid valve), rheumatic fever, hypertension, severe atherosclerosis of aorta or aortic valve ⊖
R	General cardiovascular risk factors	General cardiovascular risk factors
	• Congenital bicuspid valve • Ascending aortic dilatation	Congenital bicuspid valve
Hx	Mild-moderate: asymptomatic	Mild-moderate: asymptomatic
	Moderate-severe: dyspnoea on exertion, fatigue, exercise tolerance ↓, CP ⊖, palpitations ⊖	Moderate-severe: dyspnoea on exertion, fatigue, exercise tolerance ↓, CP, syncope

Table 81A // Left valvular heart disease

Anticoagulation strategy after valve replacement

- Mechanical valve: lifelong anticoagulation with VKA. DOACs are contraindicated.
- Bioprosthetic valve: not necessary, VKA during the first 3 mo after mitral or tricuspid valve replacement or repair can be considered
- After TAVI, patients should be started on lifelong acetylsalicylic acid in case the patient isn't yet on anticoagulant drugs.

See the Pocket *Cardiology and Vascular Medicine* for more information on cardiological conditions.

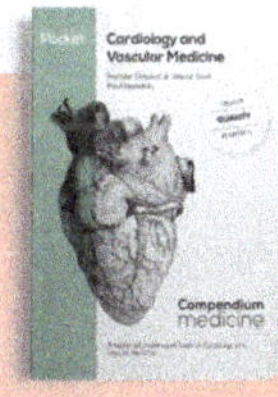

MITRAL VALVE REGURGITATION (MR)	MITRAL VALVE STENOSIS (MS)
Incomplete closure of the mitral valve, allowing blood to flow back to the LV during systole and resulting in LA and LV volume overload.	Incomplete opening of the mitral valve, leading to LA pressure overload.
Prevalence of physiological MR = ±70%, prevalence at age 65-74 = 6%, prevalence at age >75 = 9%	Prevalence at age >65 = 0.2%
• Primary: degenerative (including mitral prolapse), rheumatic fever, infective endocarditis, congenital, trauma • Secondary: hypertrophic/dilated cardiomyopathy, cardiac ischaemia → papillary muscle dysfunction/rupture	Degenerative ⊕, rheumatic fever, congenital ⊖
General cardiovascular risk factors	
LV/LA dilation	N/A
Mild-moderate: asymptomatic	
Moderate-severe: dyspnoea on exertion, fatigue, exercise tolerance ↓	Moderate-severe: dyspnoea on exertion, fatigue, exercise tolerance ↓, CP, palpitations, haemoptysis ⊖

	AORTIC VALVE REGURGITATION (AR)	AORTIC VALVE STENOSIS (AS)
PE	Watch for signs of HF	
	• Pulse: powerful • BP: systolic ↑/diastolic ↓ • Auscultation: diastolic decrescendo murmur in 3rd ICS, often in conjunction with systolic ejection murmur in 2nd ICS • Duroziez sign: diastolic murmur of the femoral arteries when applying slight pressure to the artery proximal to the stethoscope	• Palpation: carotid/precordial thrills, reduced slow upstroke • Auscultation: systolic murmur (crescendo/decrescendo) in 2nd ICS, sometimes radiating to the carotids, S4 if extreme LVH
Dx	Echocardiography and Doppler: abnormal valve shape/movement, backward flow during diastole, LV end-diastolic volume ↑	Echocardiography and Doppler: abnormal valve shape/movement, aortic valve area ↓, increased velocity across valve, concentric LVH
Tx	Wait-and-see: mild-moderate valvular heart disease/poor surgical candidate	
	Vasodilators, inotropes in poor surgical candidates/patients awaiting surgery Valve repair or replacement if: • Severe, symptomatic AR or • LV dysfunction/dilation or • Severe aortic dilation	Treat hypertension, diuretics for poor surgical candidates/patients awaiting surgery with fluid overload • Valve repair or replacement for severe symptomatic AS in good surgical candidates without contraindications • TAVI with severe, symptomatic AS in poor surgical candidates and/or (usually) patients aged >75 • Balloon valvulotomy for children or poor surgical candidates with haemodynamic instability/as a temporary solution while awaiting valve replacement/TAVI
P	• Mortality of severe, symptomatic regurgitation: 10-20% per year • Perioperative mortality of isolated regurgitation : 1-4%	• AS is the most likely valve defect to require surgery • 1-year survival rate after TAVI: 60-95%
!	Risk of HF and arrhythmias (mainly AF), increased risk of infective endocarditis and thromboembolic complications after valve replacement	

Table 81B // Left valvular heart disease

MITRAL VALVE REGURGITATION (MR)	MITRAL VALVE STENOSIS (MS)
Watch for signs of HF	
• Pulse: normal-powerful • Auscultation: holosystolic murmur at apex radiating to left armpit (more evident with manoeuvres causing preload ↓), S3 (in dilated LV)	Auscultation: loud S1, diastolic murmur with opening snap followed by presystolic murmur over the apex (no presystolic murmur without atrial kick)
Echocardiography and Doppler: abnormal valve shape/movement, backward flow during systole, LA dilation, LV dilation, pulmonary artery pressure =/↑	Echocardiography and Doppler: abnormal valve shape/movement, valve surface ↓, increased velocity across valve, pulmonary artery pressure =/↑
Wait-and-see: mild-moderate valvular heart disease poor surgical candidate	
• Acute MR: afterload reduction with nitrates, diuretics • Chronic MR: ACE inhibitors, beta blockers, spironolactone for poor surgical candidates/patients awaiting surgery • Acute MR: valve replacement for severe symptomatic mitral regurgitation • Chronic MR: valve repair, replacement or transcutaneous edge-to-edge repair (TEER) if poor surgical candidate in severe MR for 1 symptomatic patients, 2 LV dysfunction, or 3 symptomatic AF/pulmonary hypertension secondary to MR	Diuretics, beta blockers, digoxin, calcium channel blockers for poor surgical candidates/patients awaiting surgery • Percutaneous mitral balloon commissurotomy • Valve repair/replacement for symptomatic, moderate/severe MS, risk of embolism, or haemodynamic decompensation ↑
Poor prognosis in chronic, ischaemic MR	• 5-year survival rate of severe, symptomatic MS without intervention: ±44% • Perioperative mortality: 3-10%
Risk of HF and arrhythmias (mainly AF), increased risk of infective endocarditis and thromboembolic complications after valve replacement	

Dermatology

PASS ONE is a mnemonic used to describe the morphology of dermatological pathology. It stands for:

- **P**lace
- **A**rrangement
- **S**ize
- **S**hape
- **O**utline
- **N**uance/colour
- **E**fflorescence

See the Pocket *Dermatology* for more information on dermatological conditions and the PASS ONE method.

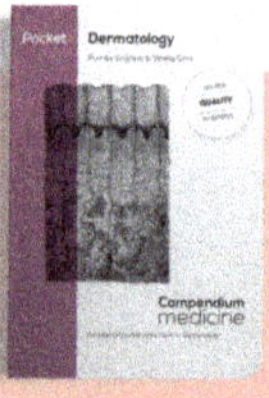

Bacterial infections

	CELLULITIS	ERYSIPELAS
D	Cellulitis is an infection localised deeply into the dermis and subcutaneous tissue, most often caused by *Streptococcus pyogenes* or *Staphylococcus aureus* (see Figure 33).	Erysipelas is an infection of the dermis and lymphatic vessels caused by *Streptococcus pyogenes*.
E	Incidence 200:100,000 patient years	Incidence 249:100,000 patient years
Ae	• Micro organisms enter the dermis through skin defects • Hematogenous spread • Portal of entry, for example between toes by tinea pedis	
R	DM, peripheral artery disease (PAD), IV drug use, immunodeficiency, alcohol abuse, lymphoedema.	Children, ♂, elderly, decreased immune function, lymphoedema, chronic ulcus cruris
Hx	• Fever, cold chills, fatigue, regionally swollen lymph nodes • Warm, oedematous, painful skin	
		Nausea/vomiting

Table 82A // Bacterial infections

	CELLULITIS	ERYSIPELAS
PE	Fever	
	P Head- and neck area in children, limbs in adults A Solitary S Single, size depending on disease progress, regional S Varies O Blurred and flat edges, subcutaneous swelling/oedema N Red E Erythematous macules, in severe infections sometimes vesicles pustules and bullae	P Lower legs, face A Solitary S Single, size depending on disease progress, regional S Varies O Sharp and raised edges N Red E Erythematous plaques, in severe infections sometimes vesicles, bullae or haemorrhagic necrosis
Dx	When indicated: ultrasound to rule out abcesses or DVT, CT to rule out necrotising fasciitis	
Tx	AB according to local guidelines, consider AB IV when the patient is very ill or if oral treatment fails. Make sure prescribed AB is effective for *Staphylococcus aureus*.	
P	• Risk of recurrence • Complications ⊖: glomerulonephritis, subacute bacterial endocarditis, and lymphoedema	• Risk of recurrence ⊕⊕ • Complications ⊖: subcutaneous abscesses, glomerulonephritis, and sepsis
!	• Mark the infection site and evaluate progression under treatment • Think of necrotising fasciitis when the patient is extremely painful, therapy resistant, or when presented with incipient necrosis, see section *Necrotising fasciitis*	

Table 82B // Bacterial infections

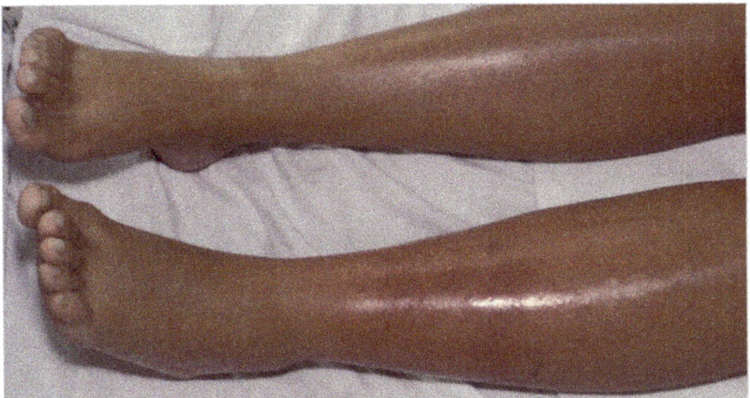

Figure 33 // Cellulitis of the left leg. The affected area is marked to assess progression/treatment effect.

Stevens-Johnson syndrome (SJS)/Toxic epidermal necrolysis (TEN)

D TEN is a rare, unpredictable, and life-threatening disease that is almost always caused by medication (80% of cases) (see Figure 34). Other rare causes are infections and vaccinations.

E Incidence 0.1-0.6/100,000 per year

Ae The aetiology of TEN is not fully understood, but is associated with an impaired medication detoxification mechanism

R Medication use (esp. allopurinol, antiepileptics, sulfonamides, oxicam, nevirapine), HIV-positive, malignancy

Hx Prodromal phase with malaise, fever, and myalgia, followed by a painful rash and blisters in later stage

PE General malaise (++), T ↑, inflammation of the internal mucosa

- P Widespread and diffuse
- A Isolated lesions, coalescent (++)
- S >30% of body surface and mucous membranes affected
- S Variable
- O Ill-demarcated
- N Redness, hyperpigmentation
- E Ill-demarcated erythematous plaques, extensive necrosis, epidermal detachment (spontaneous or due to friction)

Dx
- Lab: full blood count, electrolytes, glucose, liver function tests (multi-organ failure)
- Skin biopsy for histopathology: keratinocyte apoptosis, epidermal necrolysis and separation of the epidermis at the dermo-epidermal junction
- Consider swab for bacteriology (due to high risk of bacterial superinfection or sepsis), Mycoplasma pneumoniae serology and chest X-ray to check for pulmonary involvement of TEN, pneumonia, and interstitial pneumonitis

Tx Discontinue all potentially triggering medication, often transferred to ICU or specialised burn units

Cyclosporine or high dose oral corticosteroids

P Depends on how quickly the offending medication is stopped, mortality ±25-35%

I TEN exists as a continuum with SJS and can be classified based on body surface area involvement, with <10% being affected indicating SJS and >30% indicating TEN

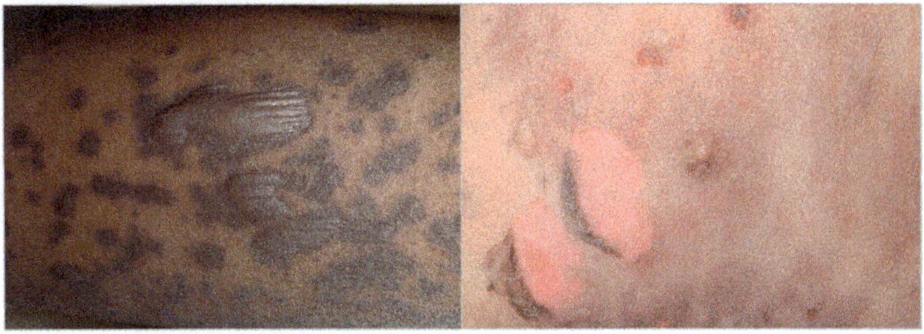

Figure 34 // Toxic epidermal necrolysis (TEN)

- SJS <10% of total body surface area and mucosa affected.
- SJS/TEN overlap 10-30% of total body surface area and mucosa affected.
- TEN 30% of total body surface area and mucosa affected.

Gastroenterology and hepatology

Ileus

D Ileus is a motility disorder resulting in delayed passage of enteric contents. Ileus is a clinical diagnosis with two subtypes: adynamic ileus and mechanical ileus (see Table 83 and Figure 35). It occurs more commonly in the small intestine (80%) than in the large intestine (20%).

Strangulation is the entrapment of the intestines (e.g. volvulus) that results in insufficient arterial blood supply, leading to intestinal ischaemia, necrosis, and perforation.

SHAVING
Causes of ileus include **s**tricture, **h**ernia, **a**dhesions, **v**olvulus, **i**ntussusception/IBD, **n**eoplasm, **g**allstones.

See the Pocket *Gastroenterology and Hepatology* for more information on gastroenterological disorders.

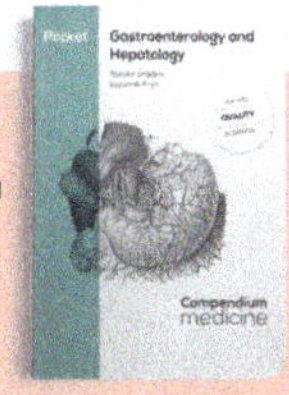

<table>
<tr><th></th><th>PARALYTIC ILEUS</th><th>MECHANICAL OBSTRUCTION</th></tr>
<tr><td>D</td><td>Ileus secondary to paralysis of the intestinal wall musculature.</td><td>Ileus secondary to obstruction of the intestinal lumen.</td></tr>
<tr><td>E</td><td colspan="2">Small intestine (80%) > colon (20%)</td></tr>
<tr><td>Ae</td><td>Paralysis of intestinal musculature → peristaltic movements ↓</td><td>Mechanical obstruction of the intestinal lumen → proximal accumulation and distal decompression of obstruction → peristalsis ↑</td></tr>
<tr><td>R</td><td>Most common causes: 6P's (post-operative, peritonitis, pancreatitis, low potassium, pelvic/spinal fracture, parturition), opioids</td><td>• Intraluminal: intussusception, volvulus, gallstones (gallstone ileus), faecal impaction, undigested food (orange-associated ileusphytobezoars), meconium, obstructive tumours (mainly in colon)
• Intramural: Crohn's disease, stricture due to radiotherapy, adenocarcinoma
• Extramural: abdominal surgery → post-operative adhesions ⊕, causing adhesive small bowel obstruction, incarcerated hernia</td></tr>
<tr><td>Hx</td><td colspan="2">Abdominal pain (persistent continuous pain with intestinal ischaemia), nausea, vomiting, absence of defecation and flatulence, distended abdomen, fever, if complicated by perforation and/or strangulation: signs of septic shock (BP ↓, heart rate ↑, clammy and pale skin)</td></tr>
<tr><td rowspan="2">PE</td><td colspan="2">Distended abdomen, hyperresonant percussion, absent liver muffling in the case of perforation, rectal digital exam reveals an empty ampulla, possibly signs of dehydration (heart rate ↑, BP ↓, turgor ↓)</td></tr>
<tr><td>Auscultation: peristalsis ↓ (ileus) or absent (silent abdomen)</td><td>Auscultation: peristalsis ↑ (high-pitched, tinkling bowel sounds)</td></tr>
<tr><td rowspan="2">Dx</td><td colspan="2">• Labs: detection of dehydration (Na^+ ↓/↑, K^+ ↓, Cl^- ↓, pH ↑), detection of infection and/or inflammation (WBC ↑, CRP ↑)
• Small intestine transit X-ray: detection of obstruction in small intestine
• In principle, the abdominal X-ray is no longer used as a diagnostic tool. If used as part of the gastrografin protocol: single dose of undiluted oral contrast is administered, followed by an abdominal X-ray 8-24h later to check whether passage is possible. There are doubts about the usefulness of this examination, but it is still in use partly due to its laxative effect.</td></tr>
<tr><td>Abdominal CT with venous contrast: diffuse dilation of all intestinal loops, no lead point, but diffuse gradual dilation of intestinal lumen, small bowel faeces sign indicating paralysis</td><td>Abdominal CT with venous contrast: lead point at obstruction site (e.g. strand, rotation, SOL), dilated bowel lumen from the lead point extending proximally, small bowel faeces sign</td></tr>
</table>

Table 83A // Types of ileus

	PARALYTIC ILEUS	MECHANICAL OBSTRUCTION
Tx	Supportive, NPO, gastric drainage tube IV fluids and electrolytes, consider total parenteral nutrition (not in the acute phase, but in prolonged ileus)	
Tx	Consider prokinetics, if possible discontinue medication with negative effect on motility (e.g. opiates) • Surgery is only indicated for treatment of underlying cause and in case of complications • Postoperative ileus: prevention is essential	• Depends on the underlying cause • Endoscopic intervention (if no signs of strangulation or perforation), stool evacuation (for faecal impaction) • Indications for emergency laparotomy: strangulation, necrosis, perforation
P	• Failure to treat ileus in a timely manner can result in potentially fatal intestinal perforation • Ileus knows a good prognosis if the underlying cause can be treated • 20-30% of patients with mechanical ileus undergo surgical intervention	
!	Complications ⊖: intestinal ischemia, perforation	• Complications ⊖: bowel ischemia, perforation, peritonitis • A prolonged mechanical ileus often develops into paralytic ileus

Table 83B // Types of ileus

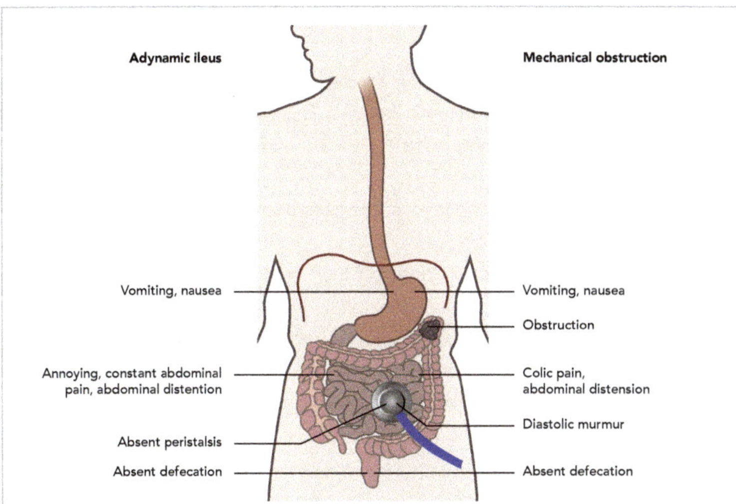

Figure 35 // Adynamic ileus and mechanical obstruction

Cholangitis

D Cholangitis is a bacterial infection of the biliary tract, sometimes accompanied by bile duct obstruction and subsequent cholestasis. The diagnosis is made using the Tokyo criteria (see Figure 36).

E ♂:♀ = 1:1, up to 9% of patients with cholelithiasis

Ae Bile duct obstruction → bile stasis → bacteria ascending from duodenum → bacterial infection

R Obstruction by gallstones, bile duct stenosis (e.g. strictures secondary to primary sclerosing cholangitis or compression by pancreatic head adenocarcinoma or cholangiocarcinoma), bile duct anastomosis (hepaticojejunostomy), obstruction of biliary stent

Hx Charcot's triad (high specificity, low sensitivity): right upper quadrant (RUQ) pain (80%), fever (chills) (80%), jaundice (60-70%)

PE
- T ↑, BP ↓, consciousness ↓, jaundice
- Features of sepsis may be present, depending on the severity of the condition

Dx
- Labs: bilirubin ↑, ALP ↑, GGT ↑, AST ↑, ALT ↑, CRP ↑, WBC ↑, blood cultures (before starting AB)
- Abdominal ultrasound: dilated bile ducts with wall thickening, cholelithiasis/choledocholithiasis
- MRCP: dilated bile ducts with wall thickening, cholelithiasis/choledocholithiasis
- Endoscopic ultrasound (EUS): to detect gallstones or sludge and as a diagnostic tool for pancreatic lesions. This procedure has no place in the treatment of acute cholangitis.
- Tokyo criteria (see Figure 36)

Tx
- AB (targeting gram-negative pathogens according to local protocol) and IV fluid in case of sepsis
- Bile duct decompression during ERCP with papillotomy, balloon dilatation, gallstone extraction and/or biliary stent placement in case of stenosis. Consider percutaneous bile duct drainage by the interventional radiologist in case of unsuccessful ERCP.

P Mortality 11-30% (in cases of severe acute cholangitis)

I Possible complications: shock, sepsis, multi-organ failure

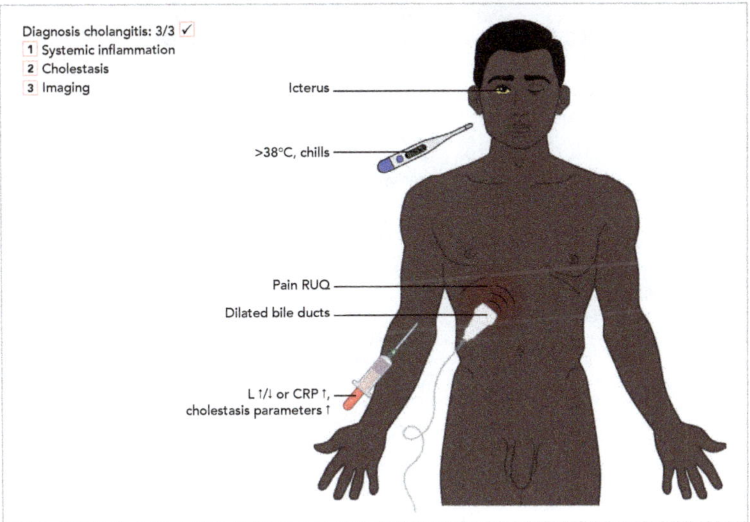

Figure 36 // Tokyo criteria for cholangitis

Tokyo criteria for acute cholangitis (see Figure 36) if I + II/III = suspicion; if I + II + III = diagnosis:

I: Systemic inflammation (T >38°C, chills, L <4 or >10, or CRP ≥10)

II: Cholestasis (jaundice or elevated cholestasis parameters and transaminases (ALP, GGT, ALT, AST >1.5x normal upper limit))

III: Imaging (dilated bile ducts (CBD >7 mm) or evidence of obstruction (e.g. gallstone, stent, stricture)

Cholelithiasis

Symptomatic cholecystolithiasis and symptomatic choledocholithiasis

	CHOLECYSTOLITHIASIS	CHOLEDOCHOLITHIASIS
D	Gallstone(s) located in the gallbladder.	Gallstone(s) located in common bile duct (CBD), see Figure 37).
E	Prevalence 15%, ♂:♀ 1:2	10-15% of people with gallstones develop symptomatic gallstone disease <10y

Table 84A // Cholecystolithiasis and choledocholithiasis

	CHOLECYSTOLITHIASIS	CHOLEDOCHOLITHIASIS
Ae	Increased cholesterol levels (in populations with western lifestyle cholesterol gallstones account for 90-95% of all gallstones), increased crystallisation tendency, decreased gallbladder motility, bile stasis (e.g. cystic fibrosis)	
R	♀, obesity, pregnancy, positive FHx, western lifestyle, rapid weight loss (e.g. after bariatric surgery), oral contraceptives, liver cirrhosis	
Hx	Asymptomatic, occasional paroxysmalepisodic attacks of severe RUQ (colic) pain due to intermittent obstruction of the cystic duct	Colic pain (urge to move), RUQ or epigastric region, nausea, vomiting, jaundice with dark urine, clay-coloured stools
PE	Not contributing	Jaundice, RUQ tenderness
Dx	• Labs: normal liver enzymes, no cholestasis, no inflammation • Abdominal ultrasound: gallstones or sludge in gallbladder	• Labs: AST ↑, ALT ↑, bilirubin ↑, ALP ↑, GGT ↑, sometimes lipase ↑ (beware of biliary pancreatitis) • Abdominal ultrasound (sensitivity 38-42%): dilated intrahepatic and extrahepatic bile ducts, CBD >6 mm (if age <70 and no prior cholecystectomy), stone shadow • MRCP (sensitivity 92-94%): dilated intrahepatic and extrahepatic bile ducts, gallstone(s) in CBD • EUS (specificity 94%): dilated intrahepatic and extrahepatic bile ducts, stone and/or sludge in CBD
Tx	• Analgesics and spasmolytics for colic pain • Laparoscopic cholecystectomy for recurrent biliary colics	• Analgesics (preferably NSAIDs), spasmolytics • Gallstone extraction during ERCP with endoscopic sphincterotomy. Consider percutaneous bile duct drainage (PTC) in case of unsuccessful ERCP (possibly with rendezvous procedure). Laparoscopic cholecystectomy is recommended <2 wk after ERCP (or PTC)
P	5-year risk of biliary colic 10%	>95% of gallstones can be removed using ERCP
!	Possible complications: cholecystitis, choledocholithiasis (if small gallstones pass into the bile ducts), cholangitis, biliary pancreatitis	Possible complications: biliary pancreatitis, cholangitis

Table 84B // Cholecystolithiasis and choledocholithiasis

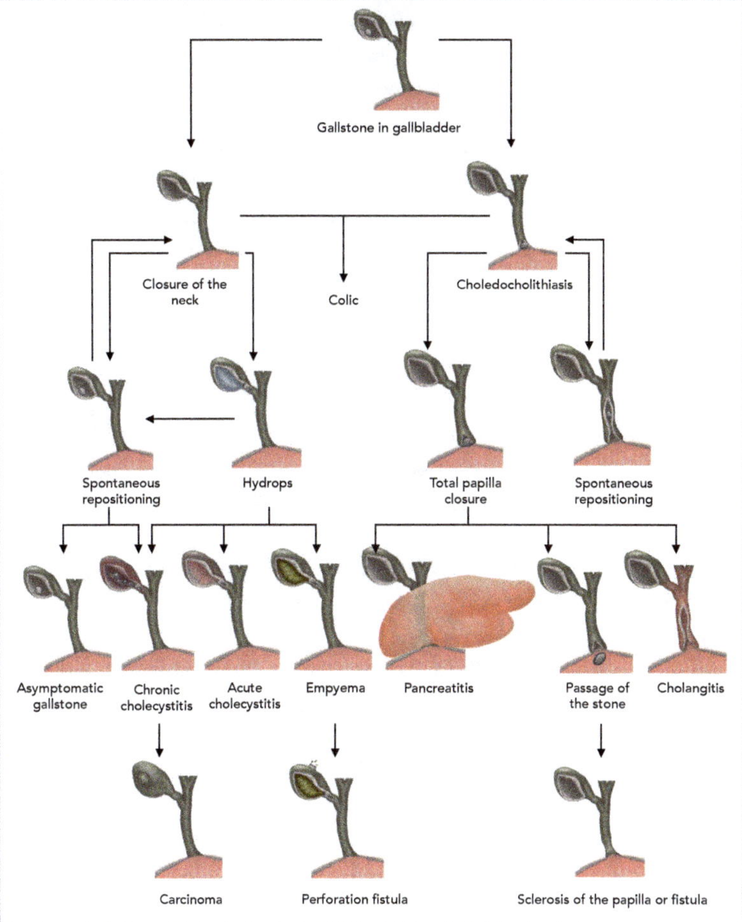

Figure 37 // Gallstone disease

Diverticulitis

D Diverticulitis is an inflammation of one or more diverticula (see Figure 38). A diverticulum is a sac-like protrusion of the colonic wall due to microperforation.

E
- Incidence 180-188:100,000 per year
- Diverticulitis occurs in 10% to 25% of patients with diverticulosis
  - Diverticulosis is present in ±60% of people over 60, ♀=♂.

- Western descent: mostly left-sided diverticulosis
- Asian descent: most likely right-sided diverticulosis

Ae Unknown, possibly faecal stasis or faecolith entrapment in a diverticulum → bacterial overgrowth → diverticulitis

R Advanced age, low-fibre diet, constipation, lack of exercise, obesity, positive FHx, smoking, use of corticosteroids use, opiates and NSAIDs

Hx Fever, lower left quadrant pain ⊕, abdominal cramps, nausea, vomiting, possible changes in bowel habits (constipation, sometimes alternating with diarrhoea)

PE T ↑, possible signs of peritoneal irritation, LLQ tenderness

Dx
- Labs: WBC ↑, CRP ↑
- When in doubt about the diagnosis or in sick patients: Abdominal CT with IV contrast (to detect diverticulitis and possible complications (covered/uncovered perforation, abscess))

Tx Depends on Hinchey stage (see Table 85) and clinical presentation

P Recurrence: 25% have complicated diverticulitis, 20% have recurring episodes <10y

! Possible complications: abscess, fistula formation, obstruction, peritonitis, sepsis

STAGE	DEFINITION	TREATMENT
0	Mild clinical diverticulitis	Wait-and-see: plenty of fluids, analgesics as needed. Indications for AB in uncomplicated diverticulitis are: immunocompromised patients, refractory symptoms or vomiting, CRP >140 or WBC >15, or fluid collection or longer segment of inflammation.
Ia	Limited pericolic inflammatory process/inflammatory infiltrate	
Ib	Limited pericolic (mesenterial) abscess	Cannot be drained: IV fluids, analgesics, and AB
II	Pelvic, intra-abdominal or retroperitoneal abscess	Abscess size amenable to drainage (>3 cm): percutaneous drainage
III	Generalised purulent peritonitis (perforated abscess)	• For Hinchey III: consider laparoscopic peritoneal lavage • NPO, IV fluids, Hartmann procedure (sigmoid resection with anastomosis or terminal colostomy)
IV	Faecal peritonitis	

Table 85 // Hinchey classification and corresponding treatment options

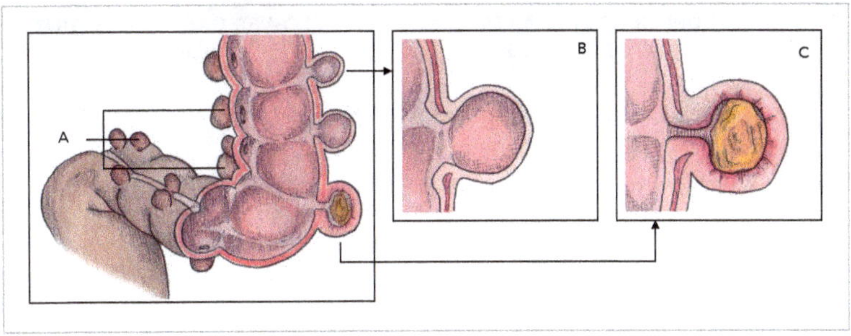

Figure 38 // Diverticulosis and diverticulitis
A: Diverticula **B:** Diverticulum **C:** Diverticulitis (inflamed diverticulum)

Gastrointestinal bleeding

	UPPER GASTROINTESTINAL BLEEDING	LOWER GASTROINTESTINAL BLEEDING
D	Gastrointestinal bleeding that originates proximal to the ligament of Treitz (suspensory muscle of the duodenum).	Gastrointestinal bleeding that originates distal to the ligament of Treitz (suspensory muscle of the duodenum).
E	Prevalence 67:100,000 per y	Prevalence 36:100,000 per y
Ae	Peptic ulcer (++), erosions (+), varices, haemorragic gastritis, Mallory-Weiss lesion, oesophagitis, duodenitis, malignancy, arteriovenous malformation (−), gastrointestinal stromal tumour (GIST) (−), angiodysplasias (−), aortoenteric fistula (−), watermelon stomach (−), haemobilia (−), Dieulafoy lesion (−), Cameron lesion (−)	Diverticulosis (++), angiodysplasia (+), cause in upper digestive system, colitis (ischaemic, infectious, post-radiation), IBD (Crohn's disease, ulcerative colitis), malignancy/polyp, rectal conditions (haemorrhoids, fissure, rectal ulcer), bleeding after endoscopic intervention
R	Depending on the underlying cause: *Helicobacter pylori* infection, anticoagulants, NSAIDs, liver cirrhosis	
Hx	Fatigue, dizziness, duration and quantity of blood loss, weight ↓, medication and alcohol use, recent surgeries/procedures in the gastrointestinal region	
	Haematemesis (bright red/dark brown), associated gastrointestinal symptoms (feeling of fullness, acid reflux, dysphagia, retrosternal pain), melaena (in case of slow upper gastrointestinal bleeding)	Melaena, haematochezia, diarrhoea

Table 86A // Upper and lower gastrointestinal bleeding

<table>
<tr><th></th><th>UPPER GASTROINTESTINAL BLEEDING</th><th>LOWER GASTROINTESTINAL BLEEDING</th></tr>
<tr><td rowspan="2">PE</td><td colspan="2">BP ↓, heart rate ↑, pallor, clamminess</td></tr>
<tr><td>Examine for underlying condition: spider naevi, palmar erythema, caput medusae sign, icterus, ascites, hepatosplenomegaly, testicular atrophy and/or gynaecomastia, epigastric guarding pain, palpable swelling tumour</td><td>• Examine for underlying condition
• Rectal digital exam: blood on the glove, palpable tumour, haemorrhoids, sometimes melaena</td></tr>
<tr><td rowspan="2">Dx</td><td colspan="2">• Depends on the underlying cause
• Labs: Hb =/↓, MCV ↓
• Labs (depending on the underlying cause): rapid blood count (e.g. Hb from venous blood gas analysis), blood group, rhesus factor, cross blood, potassium, urea, renal function, AST, ALT, ALP, gGT, bilirubin
• If indicated: lactate, CRP, troponin, CK, INR, ECG, chest X-ray</td></tr>
<tr><td>Gastroscopy: identification of the bleeding location
• In massive bleeding or haemodynamic instability, perform gastroscopy following patient stabilisation
• In haemodynamically stable patients with non-threatening bleeding, gastroscopy <24h if clinically relevant

CTA: may be considered in manifest upper gastrointestinal bleeding where endoscopy is inconclusive, or in haemodynamically unstable patients, to identify the underlying cause and location</td><td>• Haemodynamically stable patient with persistent blood loss: colonoscopy after appropriate bowel preparation
• CT angiography in haemodynamically unstable patients, possibly followed by selective angiography with embolisation</td></tr>
<tr><td>Tx</td><td colspan="2">• ABCDE approach
• Fluid challenge, for shock secondary to bleeding, consider the local protocol and possibly treating shock
• Stop anticoagulants/antiplatelets if possible, anticoagulant reversal if applicable
• Treat the underlying cause
PPI IV in suspected ulcer-related bleeding (e.g. pantoprazole bolus 80 mg followed by perfusor 8 mg/h), vasoactive medication (e.g. octreotide 50 mg bolus followed by perfusor (25-50 mg/h) for 5d) in suspected variceal bleeding, AB prophylactically only in cases with liver cirrhosis and ascites
Endoscopic haemostasis, interventional radiology, surgery</td></tr>
<tr><td>P</td><td>10% in-hospital mortality</td><td>4% in-hospital mortality</td></tr>
</table>

Table 86B // Upper and lower gastrointestinal bleeding

Hepatic encephalopathy

D Hepatic encephalopathy is a reversible neuropsychiatric syndrome, caused by metabolic changes resulting from severe hepatic insufficiency (see Figure 39).

E 30-40% of patients with liver cirrhosis

Ae Hepatic cell damage (acute/chronic) liver insufficiency, portosystemic collateral circulation and eliciting factor (haemorrhage, sedatives, infection) degradation of toxic substances ↓ ammonia (NH_3) ↑ excessive conversion to glutamate ↑ gamma-aminobutyric acid (GABA) activity ↑, cerebral oedema, oxidative stress, changes in blood-brain barrier coma

R Combination of severe liver failure, extent of portosystemic shunting and triggering factors (digestive system bleeding, infections, constipation, dehydration, medication)

Hx Various stages of loss of consciousness (confused → somnolent → soporose → coma), hyperventilation (tingling around the mouth and in the fingers, feeling of light-headedness, increased RR), West Haven criteria for grading hepatic encephalopathy

PE
- Altered GCS, changes in character, intellectual disorders (memory loss, disorientation in time, place and person), apraxia, flapping tremor, hyperventilation, Cheyne-Stokes breathing, hepatic foetor
- Depends on severity (West Haven criteria, see Table 87), possible jaundice, stigmata of liver cirrhosis

Dx
- NH_3^+ ↑ (only if indicated (!), clinical diagnosis), brain CT without contrast: to rule out other causes
- Labs: liver function tests, basic metabolic panel

Tx Symptomatic support, treat precipitating factor (i.e. GI haemorrhage), ICU admission

Lactulose (oral and/or rectal, depending on grade), consider adding rifaximin in case of recurring episodes, avoid morphine or sedatives

Liver transplantation

Lactulose is prescribed for hepatic encephalopathy. Lactulose inhibits the intestinal production of ammonia and results in an increase of faecal excretion of ammonia.

STAGE	TREATMENT
0	No confusion
1	Slight confusion, euphoria/anxiety, concentration ↓, changes in sleeping habits, irritability
2	Lethargy/apathy, disorientation to time and place, personality changes, inappropriate behaviour, apraxia, tremor
3	Somnolence, responsive to stimuli, confusion, disorientation to time and place, bizarre behaviour, speech disorder
4	Coma

Table 87 // West Haven criteria for grading hepatic encephalopathy

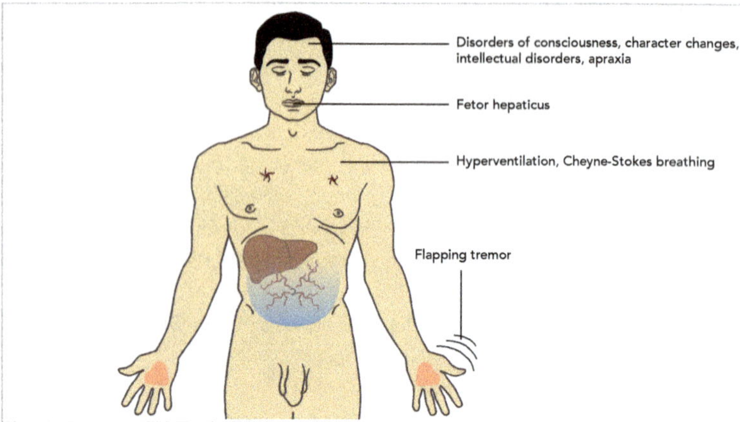

Figure 39 // Hepatic encephalopathy

Oesophageal perforation

D An oesophageal perforation is a perforation of the oesophagus (gullet).

E Unknown

Ae Iatrogenic ⊕ (complicated endoscopy), trauma, ingestion of foreign body, invasive oesophageal cancer, frequent forceful vomiting (Boerhaave syndrome)

R Endoscopy ⊕, trauma, oesophageal cancer, vomiting

Hx Depends on the underlying cause; (sub)acute (<24h) retrosternal pain ⊕, dysphagia, vomiting, hoarseness, odynophagia, beware of symptoms of septic shock